AYAHUASCA FOR BEGINNERS

Ultimate Guide to Understanding Ayahuasca and the Healing Powers of the Ancient Plant Medicine

By
Naomi Harper

Copyright 2019 by Naomi Harper - All rights reserved.

This book is provided with the sole purpose of providing relevant information on a specific topic for which every reasonable effort has been made to ensure that it is both accurate and reasonable. Nevertheless, by purchasing this book you consent to the fact that the author, as well as the publisher, are in no way experts on the topics contained herein, regardless of any claims as such that may be made within. As such, any suggestions or recommendations that are made within are done so purely for entertainment value. It is recommended that you always consult a professional prior to undertaking any of the advice or techniques discussed within.

This is a legally binding declaration that is considered both valid and fair by both the Committee of Publishers Association and the American Bar Association and should be considered as legally binding within the United States.

The reproduction, transmission, and duplication of any of the content found herein, including any specific or extended information will be done as an illegal act regardless of the end form the information ultimately takes. This includes copied versions of the work both physical, digital and audio unless express consent of the Publisher is provided beforehand. Any additional rights reserved.

Furthermore, the information that can be found within the pages described forthwith shall be considered both accurate and truthful when it comes to the recounting of facts. As such, any use, correct or incorrect, of the provided information will render the Publisher free of responsibility as to the actions taken outside of their direct purview. Regardless, there are zero scenarios where the original author or the Publisher can be deemed liable in any fashion for any damages or hardships that may result from any of the information discussed herein.

Additionally, the information in the following pages is intended only for informational purposes and should thus be thought of as universal. As befitting its nature, it is presented without assurance regarding its prolonged validity or interim quality. Trademarks that are mentioned are done without written consent and can in no way be considered an endorsement from the trademark holder.

Disclaimer

This book is intended for informational purposes only. People wishing to drink Ayahuasca should consult their medical doctors before engaging with this medicine. The use, possession, and trafficking of Ayahuasca are illegal in many countries, and the author doesn't condone the breaking of the laws of any country.

TABLE OF CONTENTS

Introduction 1
Chapter 1 *What Is Ayahuasca* 2
Chapter 2 *Origin Of Ayahuasca* 9
Chapter 3 *History Of Ayahuasca And How It Became Known In The West* 15
Chapter 4 *How To Make And Prepare Ayahuasca* 22
Chapter 5 *Uses Of Ayahuasca* 28
Chapter 6 *How Is Ayahuasca Is Traditionally Administered* 35
Chapter 7 *Different Uses For Ayahuasca And Why One Would Choose A Certain Use* 41
Chapter 8 *The Science Behind Ayahuasca* 49
Chapter 9 *Effects Of Ayahuasca On Body, Brain, And Consciousness* 55
Chapter 10 *Controversies Around Ayahuasca* 62
Summary of the Book 67
Thank You 69
Description 70

INTRODUCTION

The origin of ayahuasca has been a mystery to most researchers around the world. So many of the researchers wonder how it was possible to discover the synergy which is found in the components used when coming up with ayahuasca brew.

In this book, you will be able to learn about the meaning of ayahuasca, its history, and origin, how ayahuasca came to be known in the western countries and also how ayahuasca is prepared until it becomes ready for consumption. This book will give an explanation about how ayahuasca was traditionally administered to its brewers in order for them to take the required precautions before brewing it. It also discusses the uses of ayahuasca and why one would choose to use it for a certain purpose.

You will be able to learn about the side effects of ayahuasca and the precautions that you should take before taking it. This is meant to ensure that one does not get any health complications as a result of taking ayahuasca. There is also a chapter that discusses the science behind the use of ayahuasca and its effects on one's body and brain as well as one's consciousness. There is also a chapter that will discuss the controversy about ayahuasca and how its mystery has so far been solved.

This book is a very interesting one as it gives the reader a great insight about all the facts about ayahuasca, its benefits and also its side effects. It discusses all the highlighted things in details which enables the reader to be able to gather some knowledge about ayahuasca.

CHAPTER 1
What Is Ayahuasca

Ayahuasca is a brew which is made for a vine known as banisteriopsis together with some other ingredients. This kind of brew is made for the purpose of being used in the traditional ceremonies organized for spiritual cleansing. It was normally used by people living in the Amazon Basin. It is also used in South American and also in Brazil. Ayahuasca is normally used by many people around the world as a sacrament that is so treasured. Most of the people in the past used Ayahuasca for the purposes of spiritual connection but in the modern-day, people use it for many other purposes which include healing one's mental and physical health.

Many people have used it and have proven that it works perfectly even though there are those that it affects negatively. Such people should use it with caution since it is said to have some cardiovascular effects on them. It may increase their heart rate and in other people it may, they may experience diastolic blood pressure. People are advised to be cautious when doing this in order for them to be able to avoid heart failure as a result of taking Ayahuasca.

Ayahuasca can also have other side effects which are known as psychedelic effects. These effects are said to be visual and stimulation of the auditory system. There can also be mixing of the healing modalities as well as the psychological system which is said to cause elation and fear or even illumination. These effects are said to make people vomit and have diarrhea. When one has diarrhea or vomits, it is said to clear all the parasites and any worms in the body. They are ejected from the body when one is experiencing motility of the intestines which are said to be caused by the alkaloid.

There are people who relate dietary taboos through the use of Ayahuasca. It is believed that taking Ayahuasca makes people pure. They make sure that they remain pure through avoiding spicy as well as seasoned foods, avoiding foods which have excess fats and salt and even caffeine and any acidic foods. They also avoid sex before the occasion and after the occasion. By doing all this, they believe that they will be pure by the end of the ceremony and also maintain purity even later.

Preparation of Ayahuasca

The vine known as banisteriopsis caapi is normally boiled with the leaves of other plants. It can be boiled together with leaves of plants such as Psychotria Viridis and diplopterys cabrerana as well as mimosa tenuiflora and many other leaves. The taste is said to vary since each shaman is mixed with different leaves.

When making the traditional ayahuasca, one has to follow the customary process which requires them to use the lower part of the chacruna leaves. They are then required to say a prayer before they continue with the process. The cleaning process is also different since the vines are supposed to be cleaned through the use of a wooden spoon. It then crushed with a mallet which is also made using wood. One has to make sure that they pound the leaves until they get fiber.

Most people normally make brews by making the brews with the plants which do not have DMT. Psychotria Viridis is normally replaced with plants such as sacred tobacco and Brugmansia. All the brews will be of different quality and the taste will also be different since it depends on how skillful the brewer of the ayahuasca is.

The quality and taste of the brew are also determined by the ingredients that have been added to the mixture. There are brewers who vary the content that is in the plant alkaloid as well as its profile which also makes them get a different end result. Brewing is also done differently so the process used also affects the final result of the ayahuasca. It may also depend on the ceremony that it is being made for. This means that as the brewers make ayahuasca depending on the occasion. It also means that there are brewers who are more skillful than the others even though they gain experience with time.

Preparation of the ayahuasca may take up to seven hours even though there are those that take more hours. The preparation part largely depends on the brewer since it depends on the amount of time they use when looking for the ingredients and also when mixing them. This means that some brewers may take less time than others. There are those who have a good speed which helps them to be able to prepare the brew within a short period of time.

However, there is a reason why the brewing process may take longer is that, after the preparation process of the plants used for brewing and mixing them together in one pot, it is then boiled in a full drum. It is left to boil until it reduces to half. At this stage, the brews are mixed together and the brewers mix them until they reduce to the required amount. The results of this process are now taken and are taken to important ceremonies such as the ayahuasca.

Ayahuasca is normally used in important ceremonies. It is also used as a much-cherished sacrament. Those who use ayahuasca in traditional ceremonies use philosophies as well as cosmologies which are normally used by indigenous people. These people include the Peruvian and also the Amazon. Traditionally, ayahuasca was mainly used as medicine.

The shamans, however, advise that people should ensure that they do not use the ayahuasca without proper supervision. They are even advised to take them in front of the shamans. They are advised to do this since the shamans believe that they can steal a person's energy from them. They believe that they can steal a little energy from them since each one of them normally has a little supply of it.

The shamans are the ones who are responsible for leading the ceremonies where the ayahuasca is brewed. They have to be patient enough because it takes the whole night. It is a rite that takes long since the brewers have to be systematic in everything that they do. Before the start of the ceremony, brewers are advised to ensure that they do not take any kind of spiced food, seasoned food and also red meat or even engage in lovemaking.

This ceremony is also said to make people diarrhea and vomit which is helpful in ensuring that they release any kind of emotion that has been built up. It also helps in ensuring that they release any kind of negative energy. This enables them to be able to have some peace of mind after the ceremonies.

The traditional ayahuasca brews are normally made from the banisteriopsis caapi even though the dimethyltryptamine and the other admixtures may vary from area to another. Caapi is from a variety of mixtures which are normally known as colors. They are said to have some varying effects and potencies as well as varying uses. Below are some of the admixtures together with their ceremonial values as well as spirits.

- **Ayahuma Bark:** This is normally referred to as the deadhead tree. It is said to help in the providence of protection to people who use it in their mixtures. It is also used for the purposes of healing one's soul loss which may have been from trauma as well as from some kind of spiritual flight.
- **Capirona Bark:** This kind of admixture is used for the purposes of cleansing as well as protection. You will be able to differentiate it from other types of trees because it has very smooth bark and white flowers. It is also a hardwood, unlike the barks of the other.
- **Chullachaki Caspi:** This type of bark is used for the purpose of cleansing one's physical body. This means that it can be of help when one wants to transcend their physical body sicknesses.
- **Luna Blanca Bark:** This type of bark is also used for protection purposes.
- **Punga Amarilla Bark:** This bark is also known as the Yellow Punga. It is said to give protection to people from the bad spirits. It is said to help in ensuring that it removes the bad spirits as well as negative energies.
- **Remo Caspi Bark:** It is a type of bark which is also known as oar tree. It is used for the purposes of chasing away the dark energies away from people.
- **Wyra Caspi Bark:** This type of bark is also known as the Air Tree. It is used for the creation of purging, treatment of gastric illnesses and also intestinal illnesses. It is also used for calming

the mind as well as ensuring that there is tranquillity in one's body.

All the above barks are therefore important since they help people to be able to handle different issues that they may be experiencing. It is important to ensure that they get advice from the shamans who are experienced in all kinds of brews in order for them to ensure that they do not take anything that may ruin their health. It is also important for people to know the types of brews that are for particular occasions in order for them to be able to honor those ceremonies with them.

The Effects of Taking Ayahuasca

There are very many people who use ayahuasca and are reported to have had supernatural and also experiences that were purely spiritual. They stated that they have had revelations about the different things in life and also their purpose in the world. They have also had revelations about nature and its truth as well as having a great insight on how they are supposed to live a fruitful life.

For most Christians, this means that will get to experience an awakening of their spiritual life which they consider to be a rebirth. They feel like their strength has been renewed after the revelations. There are those Christians who say that after the revelations, they always feel like they got a connection with the spiritual dimensions. Through the connections, they believe that they are able to get healing spiritually since they are connected to the spiritual dimensions which act as their guide even though they cannot be seen with one's naked eyes.

Through the experience, people are able to experience many positive changes in their lives. When they take the ayahuasca, they believe that their lives will always change for the better. There are those who vomit and diarrhea after taking the ayahuasca. This is said to help in the release of any kinds of negative energies and also any pressure and stress they may be experiencing.

Any kind of anger, stress, and depression that people may have carried in their hearts all their lives are able to be released when they diarrhea and when they vomit. There are those who are said to experience flashes all over their body. They may experience either cold or hot flashes so it depends on one's body reaction.

There are people who get affected emotionally and may also experience some psychological anguish after taking ayahuasca. The effects may be temporary but it is important to ensure that you are cautious when taking it.

Such people are advised to avoid taking it in excess as it may result in a syndrome known as serotonin. This, however, depends on the dose that one takes. There are those who are likely to experience tremors and nausea and also vomiting. Others will diarrhea or sweat and some may also experience dizziness as well as muscle spasms. All the above are caused by the harmala alkaloids which are found in the ayahuasca. The good thing is that there are no long term effects that have been reported so it's safe to say that ayahuasca is safe for use by a large number of people.

However, there were a few deaths that were reported which were not specifically as a result of taking ayahuasca. The deaths are said to be as a result of other factors that may have been overlooked. Some of them are not screening people's heart conditions which may have caused heart failure as a result of various drugs interactions. People who may be using the antidepressants are asked to avoid ayahuasca since it is said to have some great effects on the drugs which may make them not to work as they are required to.

It is important for anyone using ayahuasca to ensure that they follow all the given instructions in order for them to be able to avoid trouble when using it. They can also seek advice from the shamans who are skilled and knowledgeable about ayahuasca, its benefits and also its shortcomings. By doing this, one will be able to use ayahuasca responsibly which will enable them to avoid getting any kind of health conditions.

Ayahuasca users are also supposed to go through a health screening process which will help in ensuring that they avoid heart conditions that may come as a result of taking ayahuasca without proper instructions. Going for screening will help to ensure that they take the necessary actions before taking ayahuasca.

The responsible shamans make sure that they give guidance to brewers of ayahuasca. They give them all the information that they require in order for them to take it with the awareness that there may be consequences of taking it. They should also monitor people when they are taking the ayahuasca in order for them to be able to avoid health issues that may arise as a result of taking it.

There are shamans who very organized so they look for experienced medical staff who take care of people who may get health complications because of taking ayahuasca. It is now clear that ayahuasca has different effects on different people. This means that they will have different experiences after using it. It is therefore important to ensure that one knows the type of ayahuasca that suits them.

Benefits of Using Ayahuasca

Ayahuasca has very many benefits since it has been proven to help many people. Below are some of its benefits.
- **Brain Health**

Ayahuasca protects one's humans cells which may have been damaged because of a lack of oxygen and even when the cell survival increases. The

B- carboline which is found in the ayahuasca is said to have a protein which is useful in ensuring that there is a healthy growth of the nerve cell. It also helps in the promotion of nerve cell existence.

Through a test tube study, it was said to have some exposure to the harmine which is responsible for increasing the growth of the human neural antecedent cells. They were said to have increased the cells by 70 percent within four days. The benefits that the brain gets is being able to generate more cells in one's brain.

- **Improving one's Psychological Well Being**

Research stated that when one takes the ayahuasca, they are able to their brain capacity which in return improves their psychological well-being. When one takes ayahuasca often, they are said to have an improved mood and improved emotional stability. This is of great help to people who may not be emotionally stable since they are able to manage their emotions. Managing one's emotions is important in ensuring that one gets to interact with people without encountering any challenges.

When one is emotionally stable, they are able to avoid stress as well as depression. This is because they are able to get away from situations that may turn out to be stressful to them.

- **Treatment of Depression, Anxiety, and Addictions**

Ayahuasca has been proven to help people who may be dealing with post-traumatic depression and also those with addiction problems. This means that after the consumption of ayahuasca, they were able to lower their stress and depression levels. This enables people to be able to interact with people well unlike when they are stressed and depressed.

There are depression patients who depend on drugs for their survival. This too can be cured through taking ayahuasca. It is said to be of great help in ensuring that they do not depend on drugs since they can be able to live comfortably without depending on the drugs. This helps a lot in improvement of one's quality of life. People who experience anxiety are also advised to take ayahuasca which helps them in ensuring that they lower their anxiety levels. It is, however, important to ensure that they look for consultation before using it in order for them to ensure that they do not get any kinds of health complications.

It is, however, worth noting that ayahuasca has some side effects so it may not favor you. This means that one may need to take consultation from the shamans before they take the mixture. This will help a lot in ensuring that they do not get any health complications after taking the concoction.

The researchers have been challenged to conduct thorough research to a certain that ayahuasca is good for the treatment of given illnesses. This will help in ensuring that people take it without worrying about their health. They will also be able to help their friends and relatives who may be having health complications that may be treated through ayahuasca.

Any time one thinks of using ayahuasca, they should ensure that they have realistic expectations about the brew. Even though there are many issues that are handled by ayahuasca, there are those issues which will definitely not be treated through taking ayahuasca. Ayahuasca is also said to work for some people but it does not work for some. Different results will be achieved by different people since different bodies react to things differently.

It is therefore important for people to ensure that they have a good attitude when taking ayahuasca in order for it to give them good results. This is because it is said that ayahuasca is meant to heal its cause and not just the symptoms of the disease.

CHAPTER 2
Origin Of Ayahuasca

Ayahuasca is a brew made from an Amazonian plant which was in use for so many centuries. Researchers say that it was in use for thousands of years all over Peru and Colombia as well as in Ecuador and Brazil. It had so many names which included caapi and yage as well as anathema and mihi. There is no clear date that one can quote when tracing the origin of ayahuasca. Researchers are however certain that indigenous people were using the ayahuasca drink in the Amazon Basin before the westerners came to know about it.

There are so many stories that are told about how the ayahuasca came into use. So many indigenous people in the Amazon region are said to have been using ayahuasca form way back. The shamans in this region are said to use it for the purpose of healing and also in divinatory purposes especially in the church. There are very complex rituals which are said to surround the rituals used when ayahuasca is prepared. They had to ensure that they have all the ingredients that were required in the making of ayahuasca. They had to get the ingredients right if at all they wanted to get the best taste of ayahuasca.

The process of making ayahuasca is said to have been passed on from one generation to another by the shamans. This continued for so many years until many shamans were discovered. The shamans were, later on, spread to other parts of Peru which helped a lot in taking the services closer to the people. Those who were not aware of ayahuasca were able to learn about it and some even started using it to solve the issues that they were facing.

The shamans would use ayahuasca when conducting the healing ceremony. They would use this medication in order for them to be able to find out the cause of the illness and the treatment that was required for their treatment. There was no written record about the origin of ayahuasca until when the Spanish researchers started researching about it in the 16th century. There was some evidence that was found in a certain cup which had traces that showed the use of ayahuasca in Ecuador. The cup was said to have been in use in more than 2500 years ago.

Ayahuasca is said to have been in use in over 75 regions in the lower and also in the upper Amazon. All the indigenous tribes are said to have been using ayahuasca for that long. The religious leaders in these regions are said to have been using shamanism for over 70000 years. However, shamanism is not a religion but a way through which people use to make a connection with the spiritual world. They are said to use shamanism in order for them to connect with the realms that were said to be sacred.

Shamanic practices have been using for thousands of years. The shamans used wisdom borrowed from their models to make the traditional ayahuasca meant for healing. The healers would use the shiplap plant medicine for their healing processes. The shiplap culture is said to have had a culture which originated from the Ucayali River which was found in the Peruvian Upper Amazon which has been for shamanism and also because of the availability of plant medicine in that region.

Shipibo culture is said to have maintained its art, language and its use of the plant medicine over the years. They are the only ones who were consistent with their culture in the Peruvian Upper Amazon over the years. It is also said to have had the most qualified and experienced healers who were so good in their healing job. They were the most recognized because of their ability to handle all the diseases without experiencing any kinds of challenges. Most people in the Peruvian Amazon, therefore, resulted in visiting these traditional healers for all their healing needs.

As time went by, people from all over the world would visit the healers in Peru. Some would even settle down in Peru which resulted in marriages between the Peru people and Spanish who continued the use of ayahuasca. Even though most of them stopped using traditionally brewed ayahuasca, it is evident that it is still in use in most Spanish countries. Those who started their families in these countries were able to access the brew from their family members or from their friends and other relatives.

Many researchers found a combination of the two plants used in making ayahuasca mysterious. Ayahuasca had to be made from the ayahuasca vine together with the chacruna plant. The plants were normally collected from the jungle and were used in the making of ayahuasca concoction. It was believed that in the process of making the ayahuasca, the mixture acquired some spirits that are in energetic and which would be used when the shamans were conducting their healing procedures.

However, nobody has discovered how shamans came to learn how ayahuasca is made. No researcher has discovered how they came to learn that the two plants can be mixed together to come up with ayahuasca. There were so many trees in the Amazon rainforest that these people would opt to use but somehow, they knew the plants that they would use for making ayahuasca. They were able to discover that the leaves of a particular plant would be combined with the vines of another to come up with a drink known as ayahuasca.

Most of the shamans used to give an explanation that they were guided by the plants when making ayahuasca. They would state that their spirits would connect with the plants which helped them to find the right plants and vines to use when making the mixture. The researcher would not believe this version of the story so they continued with their research to discover how ayahuasca came into existence. The researcher, therefore, continued to look for any information about the origin of ayahuasca but they still found very little information which was not even dated.

The only valid information that they would find ways on how ayahuasca was the purposes for which ayahuasca was used for. They discovered that ayahuasca was used for the purposes of eliminating bad luck, resolving issues that may have arisen as a result of jealousy as well as envy. These healers were able to recognize the cause of certain issues so they would give a remedy for it without experiencing any challenges. They would also help people when they needed to make any important decisions in life. They would ask for advice from the spirits and would then advise those who came to seek advice from them. It is therefore believed that it is through the plant spirits that the healers were able to know the help that people needed from them.

The shamans were also able to discover thieves. They would be able to tell who stole your items and help you to be able to get them. They would also be able to help you discover who your enemies were. This would help one to try and make peace with them which would later help them to live in peace with them. People who had been bewitched also used to go to the shamans for cleansing which was believed to later help them to be able to go back to being their normal self.

Shamans also had the skills required to enable them to prescribe the medicine that one needs in order for them to be able to get healed. This was of great help to the people who had challenges with their health were able to get treatment for it at any time that they needed it. They were also able to refer their friends who had health problems to the shamans who helped them to be able to recover too. Many people, therefore, learned about the existence of ayahuasca and which helped them in dealing in so many aspects of their lives.

The shamans were said to connect with the plant spirits in order for them to be able to handle those issues. They would sense the psycho-spiritual experiences that people were going through and would address them through their skills and expertise that they had gathered over the years. They would communicate with the plant spirits which would offer guidance on what they needed to apply in different situations. Most people depended on them for solutions to their problems since they believed that they had all the powers needed to do it. They did not have any otherwise anyway since the shamans were the only available and most trusted healers that were within their reach.

The practice was however expected to be conducted by healers who were pure and who had hearts that were sincere. A sincere heart required in order for them to avoid bias and also avoid being judgmental when they are dealing with people. These spirits would not connect with hearts that were not pure. This is because they needed a very strong connection with the plant's spirits. The chosen healers were expected to conduct very complex medical issues that required a lot of expertise. The conditions included conducting surgeries which could be minor or major injuries. It was, therefore, important to ensure that the healers were qualified and experienced to handle all issues related to surgeries. Researchers state that this kind of healing through the use of plants is only found in Amazon.

All the ceremonies that were carried out in the past were said to be attended by very many spirit doctors who would use the plant spirits to heal people. The healers had to ensure that there was ayahuasca in order for the healing process to become successful. The healers had to follow every instruction to the latter in order for them to succeed in the healing process.

The westerners came to know about it ayahuasca in the 19th century even though it had been in existence before. Most researchers have had a hard time when trying to discover the origin of this great medicine which has benefited so many people. The indigenous people normally state that they discovered the process of making ayahuasca through their interaction with the plants. They state that the plant spirits acted as their guide when making ayahuasca. The drink was normally made depending on the availability of the plants required when making the mixture.

The practices in different regions were also different since the traditions were also different. Most indigenous people believed that traditional medicine was unique in its own way since its purpose was to heal diseases that even other types of medicine cannot heal. It was therefore really treasured since people believed that it was their only hope when they got ill.

The westerners would not comprehend how the indigenous people would be guided by plant spirits so they decided to study the origin of ayahuasca through scientific methods. The modern Ayahuasca researchers state that ayahuasca is a drink that was being taken even in ancient times. The date they give is dated back to around 5000 years back. They state that the use of ayahuasca has very deep roots into the past. They say that it was available in the native philosophy and also in the mythology. This means that ayahuasca was present and was in use many years ago. When writing about the origin, it's clear that ayahuasca was in existence in 300 BC and some researcher's state that it could have even been there before 3000 BC.

Research has therefore led people to believe that ayahuasca was discovered way before we could even think that it was in existence. The process of making it could be different as compared to now but the end result is still the same and it is used for the same purposes as in the past. Whenever people search for anything related to ayahuasca drink give related results. This proves that its origin is just as many researchers have stated.

The natives of the Amazon and all those that are in the surrounding areas recorded that ayahuasca has been in existence for the last 5000 years.

They also said that it has been used as a pant medicine even in the past years. This means that people were still able to use this drink to cure all kinds of ailments that are healed through the use of ayahuasca. It was also used by religious leaders in their ceremonies just as they do it today. When researchers state that ayahuasca was in use even earlier than 3000BC, it can only mean that ayahuasca was there before even before the formation of the first Egyptian dynasty. It is, therefore, five centuries older than the leadership of Sumerian king Gilgamesh. It also means that it was present ten centuries before the devices used for the purposes of ingesting the plants that contain DMT. The plants containing DMT are said to have tested positive and they were in use in 2130 BC.

There was evidence of ayahuasca existence on a pre-Colombian rock. There were drawings related to ayahuasca which were in use in the Amazon regions. Even though most researchers only talk about things that had happened like 150 years back, there was evidence that ayahuasca was in existence earlier. In the Brazilian Amazon zone, it was discovered that people had been using a vine known as Liana which was normally used for the purposes of intoxication.

There is also an Ecuadorian scientist who was said to have mentioned the use of ayahuasca in that region in 1858. In his research, he is said to have described reasons why the vine was useful. They stated that the vine was of help in enabling the shamans to be able to foresee the future. They would be able to see any battles that were being planned by their enemies, they would also use in the diagnosis of various ailments and also in determining the spells used by the magicians of those days which helped them to know the ones that they needed to use at that particular time.

They were also responsible for welcome the tourists that visited that area. They would ensure that they insured love for their spouses through the concoction made with that vine. Villavicencio is said to have taken the drink himself and he described it as the most marvelous drink he had ever taken.

Different scientists also discovered how the drink worked. They analyzed how the shamans mixed the ingredients and recorded it. In the year 1923, scientists listed some of the hallucinogens that were used in the making of the ayahuasca. Many centuries back, the use of psychoactive drugs was said to be very important since it plays a great role in the traditions and religions in South America. Even though the use of ayahuasca was more widely spread in the 20th century. There was an outburst of tourists who visited Peru and were interested in learning about the use of ayahuasca. They would go around looking for information about the process of making it, its effects and benefits.

Discovery of ayahuasca was therefore very timely in the olden days. This is because there were no hospitals or doctors that these people would go to when they were sick. They fully depended on the shamans for all their ailments. With the discovery of ayahuasca, many indigenous people found a solution to not only their illnesses but also to the problems that they used to encounter in their day to day lives. Discovery of ayahuasca was therefore very important to the people living in the place of its discovery and also to those living far from it since, in the end, they all benefited from it.

Shamans were therefore much respected as a result of the solutions they used to offer to the people. A lot of people benefited from their discovery as they were able to get solutions to so many problems that they encountered in life. They were also experienced in their healing job. They had learned the skills from shamans who were there before them who ensured that they were qualified for the job before allowing them to handle people's issues.

We can all agree that it is a great challenge when people want to preserve ayahuasca culture. This is because most people have become modernized and would want to use medicine that they feel like it is safe for them to use. They do not believe in the use of ayahuasca for treatment. Most of the people are only interested in studying its history and not necessarily practicing it. The modern society may not really understand how the medicine worked so they only concentrate on the medicine they use now and they may not be interested in using ayahuasca even though it is still in existence in most parts of the world.

Most researchers, however, feel that it would be a great idea to preserve the culture of ayahuasca. They feel that people need to respect that culture even if they are not practicing it anymore. They need to honor the discovery of ayahuasca and ensure that they respect its traditions. This is because it's a discovery that was of great help to the indigenous people who lived in Peru and other countries thousands of years ago.

Respecting the history of ayahuasca would mean respect for those who discovered ayahuasca. It would also help a lot since people would be able to preserve the history of ayahuasca in order for them to ensure that the future generation gets to learn about its existence in the past. They would be able to learn how it was used and how healing came from its use. This will help in ensuring that the ayahuasca history is preserved for many years to come. Throughout history, people will be able to get an insight into where they have come from. They are able to appreciate what they have now once they compare the present and the past.

CHAPTER 3
History Of Ayahuasca And How It Became Known In The West

It is only recently that ayahuasca has been open for use by all people. In the past, ayahuasca was used for special occasions only. It was made for use by people who were from the Amazonian communities. This is something that was strict since ayahuasca was strictly for these communities. There were healers who were known as shamans and they were the only ones who were trusted to give ayahuasca to the members of the community.

The shamans would ensure that the administer ayahuasca to the people who were qualified to take it in terms of their health conditions. they had to be careful since there are people who have health conditions such as high blood pressure and heart conditions which can cause them problems after taking ayahuasca. The shamans would administer and supervise them as they took the ayahuasca. Shamans did not have any other job so their main job was administering and supervising people as they took ayahuasca.

These shamans dedicated their lives to serving the people in their community and through their job, they gain knowledge and skills that were required for them to be able to properly attend to the ayahuasca brewers. They would ensure that they reached all the people in their regions in order to ensure that they got ayahuasca. This was of great help especially for people who needed it for special ceremonies. They were sure that they would get it without too much struggle. The shamans have to be notified about it before in order for them to be able to prepare it. This is because its preparation is a process that may take up to a day.

The shamans' position was however not assumed by just anyone in the community. It was normally inherited from their elders. The best person to take the shaman position was the one who had been helping the shamans with the job. This would help a lot in ensuring that they learn all the skills required for them to become qualified shamans. However, even before inheriting the position, they have to go through thorough training which is meant to enable them to carry out the tasks effectively. The experience on how to collect the right ingredients, their preparation and purposes were learned over the years and were passed on from one generation to another. The incoming shamans would get guidance from the shamans when gathering the ingredients in order for them to ensure that the trainees are getting the required ingredients. It was the duty of the shaman to declare that one was now qualified to become a shaman. They had to ensure that the person that is appointed to that position was ready for the hard task ahead of them. They had to be in a position to heal people without them getting any health complications.

The shamans believed that they had the ability to heal people physically and psychologically as well as emotionally and spiritually. It is this belief that made ayahuasca to become very popular in the past as people believed that they would get a solution to all their health problems from ayahuasca.

Shamans used ayahuasca for so many purposes. I have discussed some of the use of ayahuasca in the past.

- **For Purposes of Sorcery**

The shamans in the Amazon region were best known for using ayahuasca for sorcery. They would use it for purposes of attracting clients to their other businesses. The sorcery's main purposes were to make the clients buy from them and come back to buy from them again in the future. The shamans would use their powers to heal and indeed people would get healed. This made them popular over time which made them very popular. People would come from very far to get healing through the powers of the shamans.

It is, however, worth noting that there are shamans who would mislead their clients. They would give them ayahuasca which would make their health deteriorate. Some of the clients would get mental problems while others would even die. This was a bad thing since the client's hope was to get healing but end up dying. Shamans are also said to use their shamanic powers to help their clients get their partner back after breakups. They would also help those who did not have partners to be able to get them. This was a good thing for them since they would be able to finally settle down with the partners of their dreams.

- **For Initiation**

The shamans would go through the initiation process through the use of ayahuasca. They had to use ayahuasca in their ceremony because it was a much-respected drink. All the initiates would come together and brew ayahuasca since they were there for the same purpose. The ceremony would them continue and the shamans who are already initiated would offer guidance to the new initiate on ways in which they would be required to conduct themselves.

This ceremony would be announced early enough in order for the initiate to be able to prepare themselves psychologically for it. Being prepared is very important since the procedures are not really pleasant for all people. There are those who will enjoy the drinks while there are those who would be affected by the same drinks.

As they went through the initiation process, there would be drumming and the initiates were expected to go the initiator one at a time. The rest would be left taking ayahuasca as they prepared to get in for their turn. Ayahuasca helped them to be able to endure the pain they go through when being initiated. It was therefore advisable for the initiates to make a consultation about how to fit they were to take ayahuasca in order for them to avoid complicating things after taking it and yet they were supposed to go through initiation.

- **For Healing Purposes**

Ayahuasca was believed to heal all kinds of diseases in the past. Many people would, therefore, visit the shamans for them to get ayahuasca to heal the illnesses they were ailing from. The shamans would listen to them as they explained how they felt and they would be able to tell the amount of ayahuasca they needed. They would administer it to them and they wished them well in their healing process.

The shamans were expected to supervise the patients as they took the ayahuasca in order to ensure that they do not experience any side effects from taking them. There are however people who were not allowed to take ayahuasca. Most of those who were not allowed are those who had heart conditions and those with blood pressure issues. They were not allowed to take it because it would make them experience some kind of health complications that would even result in some of them losing their lives.

The process of taking ayahuasca was sometimes so interesting since after taking it, people were expected to sit in the darkness. The purpose of sitting in the darkness was for the ayahuasca to be ingested fully into the body. The shamans also had to ensure that it had given the expected results before they left.

- **Communicating with the Spirits**

Most of the shamans used to communicate with the spirits in order for them to get the permission they needed to conduct the healing process and other activities. The shamans normally used ayahuasca to conduct the ritual of commanding the spirits. This would help in ensuring that the spirits were present when they were conducting their ceremonies. Communicating with them was, therefore, an important thing since they would help them gain the powers to heal and also help their clients.

Ayahuasca was therefore used for the above purposes and it also helped in bringing different people together for the same purpose. Most of the people visiting the shamans had the same purpose. This helped a lot in giving the shamans in gaining experience in this field since they would get to handle similar cases often.

The ceremonies were also helpful in enabling people to bond as they took ayahuasca. They would share their experiences about their day to day lives. Through sharing, people would be able to soldier on without experiencing challenges since they learned that they were not the only ones experiencing life challenges. The ceremonies would also be used to uplift their spirits. They would sing and dance to different tunes all night, especially during the ceremonies. This acted as a recipe for good mood and those who had gone to the ceremony when sad would leave feeling better as a result of the engagements they had during the ceremonies.

If we were to look at its past history, we discover that Ayahuasca was in use as early as 1000 A.D. It was a bundle which was said to contain some of the ingredients used in Ayahuasca together with some other shamanic substances which would be preserved mostly in South-western Bolivia caves. Their caves were discovered in the year 2010. Christian Missionaries who went visiting Spain in the 16th century are said to have discovered that people in that region were using Ayahuasca. Most of the Christian missionaries would call this the devil's work since they had not encountered it anywhere else.

It is during the 20th century that an active chemical which is a constituent of B.caapi was given a different name which is telepathine. After being given that name, they discovered that was the same as another chemical which had already been isolated so it was named harmine. Ayahuasca becomes popular after McKenna brothers wrote about its benefits on amazon on a page known as True Hallucinations. Later on, Dennis McKenna was said to have studied pharmacology and botany as well as chemistry on everything related to Ayahuasca which they used as a thesis when doing their masters in the university.

Another researcher named Richard Evans Schultes is also said to have asked his co-worker Claudio Naranjo to go on a journey through the Amazon River in order for him to go and study everything about Ayahuasca. He was expected to study this together with the Indians. When went there, he brought with him some samples of the beverages they discovered. They did publishing which was a scientific description of all the effects it has as lively alkaloids.

There are so many modernized religions which believe in the use of Ayahuasca that has been started. The one that has become more famous is Santo Daime and Uniao do Vegetal which is normally put in a context which is animistic which is also shamanistic. This means that it is normally merged with Christianity. It is said that now Santo Daime have started many churches all over the world. All the people in these churches are believers and users of Ayahuasca.

There are also many churches which have been started in the US as well as in Europe. These churches have been started as a result of an increase in people using Ayahuasca. This means that believers of Ayahuasca have emerged in many parts of the world. This is as a result of its benefits. It has been said to help people in the cure of mental illnesses as well as physical ones. They are also said to help people to be able to communicate with the spiritual world. These are some of the reasons that have made it very popular amongst many people around the world.

In the 20th century, the taking of ayahuasca started to spread to the European and North American countries and in other parts of the world too. People were able to start the very first churches of ayahuasca in the Netherlands. There was even a file case which was against two leaders of those churches that were started. Their names were Hans Bogers who was the founder of the Dutch Santo Daime community. The other one was Geraldine Fijneman whose charges were that they had distributed some kind of substance which was controlled (DMT).

After the two of them were taken to court, no proof was found. They did not find anything that would cause people health complications as earlier stated. This meant that they had no case to answer. The court could not stop them from using the ayahuasca brews as this would mean denying them the freedom of joining any religion which was their right.

After the case, many people were able to learn many things about the ayahuasca which made them join the religion. Since then, many other religions have also been started which has made it even more popular around the world. We can, therefore, agree that the ayahuasca popularity was boosted by a great deal when the two ayahuasca founders were arrested. Since that time, researchers have come up with different styles of ayahuasca whereby some of them are not even religious.

In modern Europe and also in North America, they discovered ayahuasca analogs which are normally prepared through the use of untraditional plants. These plants are said to have the same kinds of alkaloids. An example is the seed of Syria which are used with ayahuasca vine while the DMT-rich is used to substitute chacruna. In Australia, there are some indigenous plants that were very popular in the past and even now. They are the most popular when you compare with the other modern ayahuasqueros that are in Australia.

The use of ayahuasca has grown over time and it is being used globally. Many people around the world are using ayahuasca as a result of the benefits that come with it. Western countries have not been left behind. They discovered the use of ayahuasca through some of the westerners who were said to travel to the Peruvian Amazon. They would visit Peruvian Amazon in order for them to get ayahuasca which was said to have many benefits which include healing of the physical as well as the spiritual body.

The westerners are said to have used various theories in order for them to understand the origin of ayahuasca. I have discussed a summary of the theories below.

It is obvious that when one is making ayahuasca, they have to combine two plants. They are mixed together in order for the brewer to ensure psychoactivity. Most of the psychological westerners behave differently from the indigenous ones. They both have had different ways of life since they were taking very different kinds of diets. Their ingestion of ayahuasca may also be different as a result of the different body system. The use of ayahuasca may have spread quickly owing to the benefits that come with it. Those who discovered it would spread the word to the people around them which would make them look for it too. Its existence also got to the people through trading. As they traded in between countries, they came to learn about the use of ayahuasca which they carried with them as they were going back to their countries. By doing this, ayahuasca became very popular in Western countries. Many people around the world, therefore, started using ayahuasca for the purposes of healing some of the health issues they had and when their health greatly improved, they referred other people to it too.

There are also indigenous who learned about ayahuasca through the use of a vine which is known as a Jaguar. People would chew its leaves in order for them to be able to increase their sensitivity when it came to hunting. The leaves were said to be beneficial in boosting one's immunity, clearing parasites and also helping people to be able to increase their capacity to take in more food. The westerners are also said to have adopted the use of these leaves when they discovered the benefits that come with chewing them.

Most westerners have embraced the use of ayahuasca since they believe that it is a kind of therapy. They may not come across the traditional healers to consult them on the use of ayahuasca but at least they have access to the concoction. Today's ayahuasca medicine may not be as pure as the one used in the past but it is said to still serve the same purpose. It is however important for people to ensure that the ayahuasca medicine that they are given is good for their use. This will help in ensuring that they do not get health complications after its use and also that they get the healing that they would want from the ayahuasca medicine.

After the discovery of ayahuasca, most tourists have started a trend of going to countries where the brew is in use. The main purpose of visiting this country is to ensure that they get to learn the history of ayahuasca, its purpose, and benefits. They also get to learn about the safe uses ayahuasca which may make them decide to start using it. However, this tourism has made some of the modern shamans greedy. They are said to make ayahuasca brew that is not up to standard in order for them to make money from the tourists. They are also said to use ingredients which may be harmful after consumption. This may turn out badly as it is a risk to people's health.

It is important for western tourists to ensure that they identify legit healers in order for them to be able to get the right information that they need. They should be able to acquire the knowledge they are touring to get which will help them to be able to achieve their goal of visiting the shamans. Shamans should be straight forward in order for them to be able to help people who may be in need of the ayahuasca. By doing this, they will be able to help the westerners who are new to it to understand it and get to learn how it was brewed in the past, the ingredients used and also its benefits in one's life.

CHAPTER 4
How To Make And Prepare Ayahuasca

Ingredients used in preparing Ayahuasca

In preparing the drink, the ingredients used are plants. The most common plants that people are aware of are either those that have MAOI and DMT in them. There are also other several plants used in the preparation of the drink that is less known than the two. The ingredients that are picked to make the drink mainly depend on the one who's preparing it. The preparation may also vary in terms of the consumers and for which use they are going to use it. These factors, therefore, play a huge role in the selection of the ingredients to use. Most common plants include the *Banisteriopsis caapi* vine and the *Psychotria Viridis*. These and others are discussed below.

Banisteriopsis Caapi

This type of plant is the most common and also referred to as Ayahuasca, yage, and caapi. This woody vine is the only consistent ingredient in the Ayahuasca drink. It has certain aspects and properties that make the other ingredients used to be active in the drink. The plant caapi has alkaloids; *harmala alkalois* to be precise. These types of alkaloids are the MAOIs in the plant (monoamine oxidase inhibitors. As monoamine oxidase inhibitors, when consumed, they neutralize monoamine oxidase in the stomach that allows the DMT o take its full course in the body, especially in the brain. The DMT is the major ingredient which increases the psycho activeness of the body from drinking Ayahuasca drink. This type of plant, when used as an ingredient in the preparation of the drink, brings about relaxation to the consumer because of the monoamine oxidase inhibitors that are present in the plant.

Psychotria Viridis

This is also another major ingredient in the making of Ayahuasca. This type of plant can also be referred to as the chacruna, the amiruca or samiruka in parts of Ecuador while the former is commonly used in Brazil and Peru. The chacruna in Ecuador is another type of plant that is also used in the preparation of the Ayahuasca brew, to be precise; *Diplptyers cabrerana*. This type of ingredient is mixed with the formerly discussed plant; *Banisteriopsis caapi* to make a mixture of the Ayahuasca that an effect to the consumer of being in a not so ordinary state of mind. It is believed that this type of mixture makes you acutely aware of many faculties of life that surrounds you. This can also have effects such as having a hallucination, both the visual and aural hallucinations when the Ayahuasca drink is consumed. The mixture from these two plants,

Psychotria Viridis and *Banisteriopsis caapi* have the excessively high amounts of DMT which is dimethyltryptamine.

Justicia Pectoralis
This is also another type of plant that can be used when making Ayahuasca and it is usually referred to as piri and Masha hari. The main component in the *justicia pectoralis* is the coumarin. It is the common belief of many that this specific type of ingredient has curative properties that control symptoms such as vomiting and pain among others which will be discussed later in the book. This plant as an ingredient can be mixed with any type of other plants in making the drink Ayahuasca. A warning is given when making the drink using this specific type of plant. The consumer has to take lots of water in aiding to prevent uric acid from reaching high levels in the kidney, before taking Ayahuasca that has been prepared by justice pectoralis.

Datura or Brugmansia
Other names of these types of plants are maikoa or the toe. These two are very powerful plants that cause derision when consumed in an Ayahuasca brew that has been made by them. The datura has components such as hyoscyamine, atropine, and scopolamine. In the preparation stage, care is taken by those making the drink not to put too much of this type of plant to avoid causing higher states of delusions in the consumer. Just small quantities of brugmansia are required to take Ayahuasca. In recent times, there has been an uprising trend that has been taking place of using too many quantities of the datura in making Ayahuasca brew. Those who prepare the drink in relation to this now common uprising trend are always aiming to achieve a higher state of a 'wonderful experience' of delusion by the consumer. Higher amounts of this plant make the consumer be vulnerable both emotionally and psychologically, which to many consumers is a 'wonderful experience'. The more than necessary amounts of datura may have resulted from the instant over popularization of the Ayahuasca drink, especially in the western countries where many believe that the Ayahuasca drink contain properties that cure and offer relief in an instant when consumed, thus higher amounts than necessary being used in the preparation stage of the common south America brew.

Nicotiana Rustica
Nicotiana Rustica, just from the conjugation of its name, is a type of plant that is more of the well-known tobacco. This *nicotiana Rustica* plant just contains higher levels of nicotine than found in a typical cigarette. It can also be referred to as the mapacho or the rape'. When preparing ayahuasca, nicotiana Rustica is used to increase and elevate the attention and the awareness of the consumer. It can be mixed with several other plants to make the brew such as the caapi, where this type of mixture brings about the oral enhancement of the collective ayahuasca drink to the consumer. When used, nicotiana Rustica brings about the

more lasting effect of the Ayahuasca drink, the emotional and psychological ones. There are several ways that the nicotiana Rustica can be prepared to use in the brew. Some makers of the Ayahuasca will just blow the powder form of this plant right up on the nose of the consumer when the desired results are to cleanse and purify the consumer. Another way, which is associated with the drink is directly adding the plant to the mixture of other plants making the brew. Those who make the drink in such a manner always desire for the effects of Ayahuasca to be felt at the same time. This type of plant is a difficult one to prepare and it takes an experienced hand in making Ayahuasca add and mix it in the drink to produce a brew that won't have negative and damaging effects to the consumer. Care has to be taken when making Ayahuasca with nicotiana Rustica to follow the right procedure when mixing with other ingredients to offer great curative services to the consumer.

Ways of making Ayahuasca

Preparing the brew is a long and tedious process that requires those making the drink to be careful in adding and mixing the ingredients and also patient to make the drink with its desired effects. There are several methods that can be used in preparing the brew that is discussed below and in detail. The ingredients to be used such as the datura plant or the caapi can easily be accessed from the various online outlets when not in South American countries, one such outlet common for the ingredients is the Botanical spirit. A step by step evaluation of the process of its preparation will be made and the different ways that can be employed.

The recipe of Natema

The Natema recipe is of the Shuar. The Shuar makers of the drink have a precise way of preparing the brew. Ingredients used in this method are Banisteriopsis caapi, *Diploterys cabrerana*, *Heliconia stricta*, Malpighiaceae and the *Ilex guayusa*. The first step is to split a piece of the woody vine; Banisteriopsis caapi, which is usually in a length of 1 or 2 meters. The vine is split into smaller strips of shorter length. Several liters of water is then boiled in a pot, whereupon boiling, the shorter strips of Banisteriopsis caapi are placed in the water. The second step of this method is to then add the leaves of the following ingredient plants. The *Diplopterys cabrerana, Heliconia stricta, mukuyasku,* and *Ilex guayusa*. The Ilex guayusa is a type of species of the Herrania class. The mukuyasku plant whose leaves are used is a type of Malpighiaceae. The mukuyasku is an unidentified plant of the aforementioned class of plants but still used though. The resulting mixture of several liters of water, the split strips of Banisteriopsis caapi and the leaves of the mentioned plants are boiled together up to when a mixture in a syrup kind of form is left on the pot after most of the water used has evaporated. Such type and step by step manner of preparation are also not only used by the Shuar but also the Kamsa, the Secoya and the Inga of South America.

The recipe of Caapi and *Mimosa Hostilis*
One of the main ingredients in this method of preparing and making Ayahuasca is the Banisteriopsis caapi. When making the brew in this manner, it is assumed that the caapi, when mixed with the Psychotria Viridis, results in the formation of the South America traditional brew and drink. This method is also based on the fact that the caapi plant is also majorly referred to as Ayahuasca itself as the drink and it is therefore very important to be used in preparing the traditional drink. It is assumed that the other types of plants used as ingredients are just but helpers of the caapi. This method is in preference of the caapi as the main ingredient to be used to the other plants containing DMT for the consumers view it as an ingredient with more reliable effects.

The specifications and the amounts to be used are as follows. The vine of the Banisteriopsis caapi when it is the whole woody vine, in an amount of 50 grams. The root bark of *Mimosa hostilis* plant when it is no in powder form. 12 grams of his is required. Other ingredients include white vinegar, water; distilled water. The use of stainless steel pots will also be of great import with the number required being four.

The first step is to shred the caapi with the hammer. One will have to tie the vines in clothing before the shredding. The mimosa is also ground to be in a powder form by either using the hands or a most preferred grinder. The next step is to put the powdered mimosa and a teaspoon of the white vinegar in one of the stainless steel pots. Water is then added, an approximate of one liter or so. The next step is to put the shredded caapi in another stainless steel pot, one teaspoon of vinegar and a liter of water. Both the two mixtures are allowed to boil for approximately 2 to 3 hours, up to when the water levels have decreased. The level of the heat used to boil should just be adequate such that the mixtures will just be cool enough when boiling and there will be no bubbling over. Care should be taken to ensure that there is no bubbling over. The two mixtures; the mimosa one and the caapi, should be kept separate. They are then filtered separately until they have become clear. Most commonly used filter is to use a shirt bound by duct tape.

Replace the shirt with another fresh one when it becomes clogged with the residue. The now clear separate liquids are then taken through the same process of boiling without bubbling over. More water is added to each pot another set of one teaspoon of white vinegar. The caapi and the mimosa are to be boiled for not more than three times. The resulting liquids are kept separate in different pots. When filtering for the second and the third time, low heat is to be maintained. After this process, there are two pots that each contains mimosa that has been filtered for three times and a pot with caapi that has been filtered for three times. The quantities will have been reduced by this time. The dosage of these mixtures is to be the measure of a cup at most and not less than half a cup. The mixture should then be cooled overnight in a fridge.

The next step happens the following day cooled mimosa is taken out of the fridge and filtered through yet another shirt where care is taken to prevent the disturbing of the sludge and the residue that is not wanted at this stage of preparation. This process, however, is not repeated for the caapi cooled liquid from the fridge. When this step in the process is done correctly. A liquid that is clear and one that has a purple color when it is heated is gotten. The color of the brew is more or less red like red wine. When all these steps are through, the two mixtures can be either mixed or consumed as one drink or a consumer can decide to drink one brew after another, say the caapi after the mimosa one. Because the cooled caapi was not filtered, it should be shaken thoroughly to ensure that the residues are not at the bottom of the container but rather in the drink. Before the mixture is ready for consumption, it is to be heated making it warm.

There are various points to put into consideration when making the Ayahuasca using this method. The recommended strips of the caapi plant that are to be used are the real woody vines. The real vines might cost a little bit more but the resulting brew will be worth, leaving the consumers with a 'wonderful experience'. Even though the real woody vines might be a little bit expensive, the approximate dosage of a cup of the resulting liquid is still fair in prices when the prices of other hallucinogens are put into consideration. There can also be an alteration to the required amounts in the above-discussed steps. If the mimosa is lacking, the leaves of Psychotria Viridis can be used.

The amount to be used is still the same one as that in the case of mimosa; 50 grams. When the leaves of Psychotria Viridis are used, the resulting mixture from heating without bubbling, and the addition of the one teaspoon of vinegar should not be immediately reduced when washing away the residue. The mixture should be stored in containers and cooled in a refrigerator until the next day.

The pots that are to be used in boiling the mixtures should be absolutely stainless steel and not any other material. Aluminum should not be used in any case as Teflon should also not. There is also a leeway that is given when the pots are insufficient and are not four in number. It is possible to just use one pot throughout the whole preparation stage for all the steps. On the boiling and the brewing step, both the mimosa and the caapi mixtures can be combined and boiled in one pot. The same ones from the reduction step. They can be both combined together. When this kind of preparation procedure is done, the boiling and the brewing step has to be carried out overnight for an effective brew of a drink. Only when the residue particles have settled at the bottom of the container in the fridge is the mixture to be reduced in this step of this procedure. The mimosa mixture is the only one that can be reduced in by pouring off the sediments after the mixture has cooled in the fridge overnight. The caapi mixture, however, cannot be reduced in such a manner without negatively affecting the quality of the drink since the sediments and the residue from the caapi mixture are required to be in the Ayahuasca drink. When storing the Ayahuasca in preparation for consumption, a dark, cool place is preferred as a storage place. The mixtures also have to be stored in containers and pots that are well sealed. The storage period is usually several weeks and can also extend to several months. Before the Ayahuasca is consumed from its storage, it has to be boiled each time. The type of vinegar to be used is also to be put into consideration. Only the white vinegar is to be used, not plum vinegar or wine vinegar. The use of either of these two types of vinegar can result in negative effects on the health of the consumers.

The recipe used in Ecuador and northern Peru

This is another type of recipe that is mainly used in Ecuador and the northern parts of Peru. The ingredients used in this procedure are the B.Caapi and the C.Viridis. The amounts required for the B.caapi is 50 grams. The vines that are used should be woody and fresh. The 50 grams of the caapi only applies to one person. The amount to be used for the C.viridis leaves are is 85 grams. This amount also only applies to one person. The first step is to make the strips of the caapi vines and have them between the leaves of the P.viridis plant. They should be placed in an alternate manner between the leaves of the Viridis plant. The pots used for boiling are only to be stainless steel pots or pots that are earthenware and not any other material. The mixture should also not be covered with water. The boiling time for the mixture is 4 hours, where it should be gently brewed. Afterward, the liquid is collected after it is poured off. The next step is to repeat the procedure using the same strips and leaves of the ingredients used in the fist and the second step and do away with the plant matter afterward. Both the caapi and Viridis liquids are mixed to obtain one solution which is gently boiled. The liquid should not be boiled to an extent of bubbling over to avoid loss of properties of the ingredients. A concentrated Ayahuasca drink is obtained.

CHAPTER 5
Uses Of Ayahuasca

Medical Use of Ayahuasca

There are people who have a varied reason why they use ayahuasca. Some simply want transformation or healing from the substance. It is true that some patients resolving to have the brew so as to heal. Most of the patients who have been attracted to the stimulant are those with mental health conditions. It has been witnessed by some patients ailing from depression and post-traumatic stress disorder taking ayahuasca in moments they are not satisfied with their medications. There are other people who suffer from chronic diseases such as cancer. The aim of patients who suffer from chronic ailments based on the hope of healing.

1. **Ayahuasca Curing Depression**

Ayahuasca has the potential of curing depression. This is a problem affecting several people across the world. There are several things that happen in an individual's day to day life situations that can make an individual have depression. However, ayahuasca reduces or can cure depression at an estimated time of around three to four hours after it is ingested by a person. There is a similarity that is shared between ayahuasca and other antidepressant drugs. This substance like antidepressants, it changes the serotonin concentration. Serotonin is a neurotransmitter that is responsible for boosting a person's mood.

There is also another way that this substance deals with reducing or curing depression. The substance contains a very important ingredient. The substance is commonly known as DMT which is a psychoactive chemical. The chemical is known for two effects it has to an individual's body which is the induction of revelations that have spiritual attachments and triggering the experiences an individual has. There are several people who have turned to ayahuasca. In return, they have been able to find their solace in the brew. The comfort in the substance is cemented with this person being able to get the cure they desire. However, the experience about the drug differs with people, as some have terrifying, enlightening, or both experiences.

The most common case that ayahuasca cured depression was the one shared by Kirby Surprise. It was an encounter with one of the people who used ayahuasca. It was about a man who suffered from depression because he was at a graduate school jostling between two jobs so as to provide for his family. It was a very difficult time for the person because he could be able to experience any kind of joy in his life. It was a hard struggle trying to balance work, family, and education. This made hi to resort for medical help to help manage the condition and situation. He was prescribed for several forms of antidepressants by the medics. They did not work and he was prescribed Zoloft be used for the rest of his life. However, the drug took a toll on his marriage and health life. He was not able to have an adequate or good form of sleep. It proved difficult for the guy to have a fulfilling sexual life that made his self-esteem to really deteriorate. The situation made him to even resort to talking therapy and other medicines to see if they could help him. It still did not prove to help him since he felt something was missing. His attitude towards work and his wife took a wrong turn.

The situation forced him to turn to a different form of healing. He took the initiative of studying shamanism and the medicinal plants that are involved in the events conducted by shamans. He then took another step to attending an ayahuasca conference where he was further educated. He was able to discover that the product had been used by members of UDV. The light about people who use the brew having low levels of depression being helped and changing to be social was also shared with him. There were no mental or physical side effects on an individual who was using this substance. He was also able to meet people in the conference who were long term users of the substance. These people appeared to be more healthy and sane than the people he met in his day in day out life.

A decision to use the drug was made by the man without the support of his wife. The man experienced something that was unexplainable and unimaginable. He saw lights, colors, and visions. The images he perceived were very intense and beautiful. The beauty of the intensity of the images made him shed tears. This was followed by lessons that were coming in. He was able to realize how he was losing the awareness of his body and he was treating his wife in a bad manner. The poor treatment was because of the depression he was going through. The experience was described as being scary, beautiful and painful. He was able to realize that he was so angry and cold most of the time.

The ayahuasca experience made the man feel alive again. He is able to process emotion currently and feel alive. The major feelings of love and gratitude have been the cornerstone of his life. The wife tried to awaken him the moment he was weeping and sobbing. His wife thought that he was hallucinating. However, the man told his wife that he was of his feelings at the current state. For the first time, the man woke up being filled with joy and gratitude. He could now be able to open up and appreciate his family and the surrounding.

2. Ayahuasca Curing Cancer

There are several people who have made long trips to ayahuasca centers in Peru. Their efforts were not futile because they were able to return to their hoes feeling revitalized. There are other people who have tried the drug in other places. The reports from these people have been similar to those of people who traveled to Peru.

One of the people who have visited the ayahuasca centers is known as Donald M. Topping. He was a professor from the country known as Hawaii. Mr. Donald was motivated to visiting ayahuasca centers because he was diagnosed with cancer of the colon. This was the same case to a woman known as Margret De Wys who is a writer. Mrs. Margret De Wys is a survivor of breast cancer which is one of the most prevalent forms of cancer in women. However, Margaret and Donald attended ayahuasca ceremonies in different places. Despite the difference, the result of the cure was reported by both parties. The two individuals were ascertained to be cancer-free after their experiences. The two people are just a few numbers of people who have been cured of cancer. This is because of the low levels of people who go on record. The number of people claiming to have healed from cancer after taking ayahuasca is growing year in year out.

There was a Brazilian study that was conducted by Mr. Eduardo Schenberg. He is a man hailing from the University of Sao Paulo. The study was able to establish that ayahuasca has the potential of treating cancer. The potential possessed by ayahuasca is based on the active principles that it contains. The active principles being referred to this case are harmine and DMT. The two components have high positive influence levels on cell cultures which is critical in studying cancer. This makes them very important in the biochemical process that is critical in the treatment of cancer. The importance of the substance in the biochemical process cuts across both the in vivo and vitro.

The research conducted puts a person and the globe on a different level. The new level entails people taking the reports of cancer patients getting cured in events they attend and take ayahuasca brew, this is also backed by the hypothesis elucidated above. The scientific process to prove this occurrence has undergone various rigorous tests and experiments. The reason based on intense scientific experiments is intriguing. The most important reason is to pave the way for research that will be conducted in the future that will be more advanced.

3. Ayahuasca Curing Post- Traumatic Stress Disorder

The major cause of Post-Traumatic Stress Disorder is life events that are scary and life-threatening. There are war soldiers and veterans who developed this condition. The latter turned to take ayahuasca brew for them to have relief. There are soldiers and veterans who took medicines and had a different outcome from other people. The soldiers and veteran with a different outcome reported of the prescribed medicine not changing their condition. The group later planned a visit to Amazon.

The trip was to search for a new form of cure to help then root out the condition. The trip proved to be worthwhile because they achieved their goal of getting treatments. They were able to return home in a clean state with less baggage in life and a new view of how to leave. The leaves and vines used to make ayahuasca helped the group with several things that helped them experience quality life again. They were able to wash away suicidal thoughts, combat mental pain, and bitter experiences. These were some of the factors that were holding the soldiers back to achieving their set out and planned life.

There are several people who seek to know how ayahuasca cures Post-Traumatic Stress Disorder. The substance has the potential of opening an individual's subconscious part of the brain. This is an important thing that helps patients suffering from PTSD to conquer the ailment. The brew goes a notch higher to reprogramming an individual's brain. This is done through reorganization and neutralization of the environmental symptoms and triggers of Post-Traumatic Disorders.

Another factor that ayahuasca does that makes it possible for people suffering from this mental disorder experience healing is also present. It brings the memories of the traumatic event from the subconscious to the conscious part of the mind of an individual. This makes the memories to be easily processed and make them be integrated into an individual's life has a deeper meaning. It makes it easy for an individual not to handle the emotions presented when the event replays in an individual's brain because it is accompanied by a low amount of intensity. It is why patients who suffer from Post-Traumatic Stress disorders are able to develop a better perspective on the thoughts and things that used to torment them.

4. **Expansion Of The Conscious**

Expanding an individual's conscious is one of the functions tasked to ayahuasca brew. This action is dependant on the experiences that are known to a person along to his or her conscious capacity. The resulting impact of this act is very beneficial to an individual. It helps an individual who looks to expound his spiritual, life and relationships fulfillment. There are two events that ayahuasca process does to an individual to make the fulfillment a success. It opens a person to get a better sense of knowledge to understand the mental process. It also helps in the revelation of a deep understanding of certain situations.

The overall experience of an individual makes him or she have a difficult for an individual to avoid other realities life presents an individual. They also have the potential of making a person increase his or her level of awareness and they allow one to meet his or her thinking process in completion. What the brew is able to do at a psychological level is supposed to be keenly looked at. The substance enhances an individual's perceptions and feelings which makes an individual's reaction, self-reflection, beliefs and thinking to be more vivid with high intensity.

There are several people who enjoy the experience ayahuasca brings to an individual. One of these people is known as Russ Binickii. He is a soldier who was able to survive the war which was experienced in Vietnam. The experience the Vietnam War brought to him was very traumatic. He lost two of his closest friends in the battle. The events went even to him experiencing several plane crashes which were caused by mechanical failure. When he was from war, he engaged himself in self-destructing behavior. He used to smoke pot, engage in fights and drinking. These actions placed him to dangerous spots since they were being used as the coping mechanisms for the high-intensity experiences he encountered in Vietnam.

Mr. Russ was always in a denial state of his anger state and Post-Traumatic Stress Disorder condition. He could get angry in a spur of a second. The anger state would get triggered with small things. This made him angry while driving, at home, at home, during social events or even while on duty. Russ could get angry in moments even his children would get home late past the agreed curfew time. The condition sent him to use ayahuasca because he saw it getting worse. He arranged to travel to Peru which made his life have a complete turn. Learning more about himself and his behaviors were the critical part of his transformation. Russ was able to accept his anger related problems which gave a platform to better him. The platform gave him the strength to confront bad thoughts using a different perspective.

Mr. Russ describes his anger to be triggered by guilt. He was devastated after losing three of his friends in the Vietnam War. It felt really bad to him having left without his deceased friends. It was because he was able to see his friends lying lifeless on the battlefield. This was the reason that made him be strict of curfew he put on his children. The Vietnam War rewired his brain to think that if anyone got late past the curfew time meant that he or she was in trouble. The same paranoia and panic could strike him any time his daughters were late. Ayahuasca proved to improve an individual conscious and making him change his behavior.

Ayahuasca is commonly referred to as a healer because of the inner functions that it has. They make an individual experience the spiritual and psychosomatic shifts. The functions go a notch higher to initiating physical changes and the shift from addictive habits that are self-destructive. The experience inspires users and makes them work so hard to bring a change in their own lives. The process brings about genuine change in an individual's life, allows legitimate transformation and makes the process of self-healing viable. A deeper look into an individual's beliefs, ideas, realities, and ideas are points where the healing effects of ayahuasca hail from. The potential contained in ayahuasca helps an individual gain supportive knowledge about him or herself. The process is effective because the substance tries to deal with the problem internally.

Spiritual Use of Ayahuasca

There is a major role that ayahuasca plays to spirituality. It is described as a spontaneous teacher in this field. This is despite the presence of phenomenological status describing the source not being available. There are certain important aspects that an ayahuasca practitioner possesses. He or she has the ability to gain strong insights and revelation that he or she can guide people. It is very helpful when an individual wants to bring the individual who is interested in learning or understanding the ceremony. Ayahuasca will make it possible for a person to open other human being neuro-paths that gives an easy channel to making learning to be swift. Ayahuasca simply makes it easy for a person to experience a deep divine connection with the supernatural world.

The brewed substance known as ayahuasca is very popular in helping in spiritual health improvement. It is a substance that has been in various religious ceremonies. It has been referred to as the vine of the soul. This has been confirmed by Sita who is an ayahuasca user since it affected her spiritual and emotional experience. It was able to massively change the perceptions and perspectives that she had. The process was able to make her have the most challenging bliss emotionally. Sita considered the process to be spiritual. This was because she was choosing to seek the meaning of her life and how to surrender. What the process revealed to her several sources of creation. This put her to a point of realization that there was a supreme being that had supernatural powers. Some people would prefer the supernatural being as God, Buddha or Allah. Despite different beliefs, there was a supreme being controlling the universe.

There are other people who used ayahuasca brew that have a different experience from it. They believed that they had died and resurrected again. There are a group of people that felt that they had had a connection with the divinity which some went t levels of saying they had seen God. Understanding humanity and finding the connection to it is another great purpose served by ayahuasca. There is always a powerful explanation behind the source of everything in the world. People who seek spiritual experience try to explain the experience use ayahuasca as unexplainable and unimaginable. It made them have some alteration of how they perceive the sacredness and purpose of life.

There have been studies to prove this phenomenon brought about by ayahuasca. The study proved that ayahuasca has the potential of improving an individual's spirituality. Another study was conducted on ayahuasca and those who use it. The study was able to reveal that people who are frequent users of the brew had impeccable points when it came to Spiritual Orientation Inventory. These people also passed in the other nine components that were tested. The nine components included tests in fruits of spirituality, transcendent dimension, mission in life, meaning and purpose of life, tragic awareness and sacredness of life. The points attained by people who regularly used ayahuasca still remained high on the board even after taking the second assessment that was conducted. The tests were a positive affirmation that ayahuasca brew is very important in improving an individual's spiritual health.

CHAPTER 6
How Is Ayahuasca Is Traditionally Administered

The Amazon people first and very importantly, use ayahuasca as a preservation of their heritage and identity. This is what makes this community known all over the world. There are no other people active in their herbal medication as the locals from Amazon. Therefore traditionalists who are the witchdoctors make sure they make the best brews for tourist attraction. People from all over the world travel to countries like Peru, to get this famous brew of Ayahuasca, which is used as traditional medicine. Many people are adopting the idea of using traditional medications because they are said to be the safest and most effective medication. Due to its popularity, this has seen a lot more people continue believing in it more than other types of medication. Not only is it complex to understand, but it is also very powerful. For this reason, tourists are attracted to it and want to learn more about it. It is from this that they get to learn of its benefits and therefore make use of it in making the modern medication.

Due to the numerous tourists, this brew attracts, Ayahuasca is administered along with other plants to create the better medication in the modern world. The traditionalists, along with the doctors, are teaming up to get more ways of using this popular plant. It is through the popularity of this plant among the traditionalists that the doctors have started believing in its effectiveness. If carefully studied, the plant may create ways for more effective medications. It may create a cure for diseases that are feared so much in the modern world. The herb is so popular that it has even introduced tourism to the locals. Most tourists will travel to South America just for the herb. This has helped the economic growth of the locals so much. Thus most locals have invested their time and resources to farm this plant. It is especially favorable for the locals who wait on the tourists because; importation of the substance in some countries is illegal. Therefore people who have heard about its great effectiveness and would want to try it have to travel all the way. Due to how much it takes charge of the brain, it is usually considered as drugs and thus the reason why it is deemed to be illegal in most parts of the world. It is argued that if it has the kind of effect, it does when used as a drug; it would lead to many deaths. This is somehow true because a number of people have died after consumption. However, the witchdoctor's advice the tourists coming in from time to time to consume it only with a highly knowledgeable witch doctor around. The same goes for the locals, they may grow the plant, but before the consumption of the substance, there has to be the presence of a witchdoctor. This is done to protect people in case anything goes wrong. It is so risky because ordinary doctors would find it hard to treat a person under the effect. The witchdoctors, however, due to their experience in handling the substance know the remedies and can easily administer first aid.

Ayahuasca is mostly used as a spiritual medicine that helps people reaffirm themselves or what is modern-day called meditation. It is very useful for connecting people with their spirituality because of the effects it has on the brain. Ayahuasca has substances that make someone want to open their inner selves and connect with something greater than themselves. When feeling stressed, Ayahuasca is used to help relieve the stress and therefore, a great way of reaffirmation. It helps people forget their numerous problems, even just for a while. It also helps to treat depression cases among the locals. People going through traumas also use the substance to help them overcome the difficult times. This could be mainly because the substance takes over the person by making the brain stop the normal functioning.

Ayahuasca is shared among the Indians, and they mostly use it for their rituals because it helps them with the ritual activities such as dance and songs. Religious leaders in the tribes also use it as a sacrament to the people. Traditionally it is also administered as medication. When consumed, it has an effect on the conscious thirty minutes after it's used. It then starts to raise the effects more after two hours. The effects last for as long as six hours, depending on the person that has consumed the medication.

Ayahuasca is also used traditionally as dieting recipe. It's believed that when consumed, it helps a person abstain from spices, fats, and any acidic foods a person may want to avoid. It's also used to help lower the urge for sex so that a couple is able to wait until the marriage ceremonies. The witchdoctors, however, discourage the usage of ayahuasca when a person is not near an experienced witch doctor. This is because the effects are too complicated for ordinary doctors to handle

Ayahuasca is taken as a tea to help people strengthen their feelings. How this is possible is because it's like a drug, and it makes someone high just as a drug would. When one is feeling high, the Amazon people reason that that's the best time to get rid of the bad emotions and replace them with positive feelings. The Amazon people believe that you can be anything you want to be when the tea has taken over you because it's almost as if you're reaching the greater being. It is said that the brew takes you into the other world where you get to meet the ancestors who in return, take over your feelings. This is almost the same as hallucinating, but the Amazon people strongly believe in this and therefore regularly use to reach the other side of life.

The amazon people believe that Ayahuasca is a wisdom plant. And they, therefore, believe that by consuming it, one will be wiser than they were before. For this reason, the plant is much used by the people here of all age groups. The young and the old all go for it so that they may gain wisdom. The dosage, however, varies depending on the person taking it due to its high strength. The understanding they believe is from the ancestors because they believe the plant to be a blessed tree. Rituals were done using the plants, and therefore they think that when you use it, you inherit some of the ancestor's wisdom.

Therefore for settling issues within the community, the Ayahuasca plant is consumed by the elders. When they drink it, they get the wisdom to resolve the discrepancies amongst the people. They believe that it is the ancestors that help them sort the issues since they know the whole truth. There is no issue that cannot be settled by the elders because they feel that the ancestors will help them solve the problems. Men who are about to be inducted into elders of the community are made to consume it as it will give them the wisdom needed for elders.

Since it is also used for rituals, Ayahuasca is believed to be an excellent source for learning the secrets of the other world. Whenever the people have calamities and do not know how to interpret them, they call the witchdoctors. The witch doctors then perform rituals that connect them with the ancestors who help them understand the disasters they are going through. Therefore whenever they have issues like drought or anything that is beyond their understanding, they will use the plant to contact their ancestors. They also believe in keeping in touch with their ancestors so that they can be guided in their daily lives, and the way through which the ancestors communicate to them is only if the elders perform rituals. Ayahuasca is used as a pathway to reaching the other side of their spirits, without which, there would be no connection.

Smaller portions of the substance are used to help with the treatment of other illnesses like stomach problems. It makes a person throw up and get rid of any harmful food in the stomach. It helps eliminate anything harmful in the body and is believed to be a blood cleanser. It is, however, not very recommended for regular users because it has a lot of side effects both for the body and the mind. However, the locals believe that when it is proper prevention for minor illnesses. Diarrhea and the throwing up will prevent any poison from staying in the stomach. Diarrhea resulting from this substance consumption, however, is so severe and could lead to death. The locals don't seem to mind this, however, and neither do the tourists who keep flocking in to use it. It all goes down to how much a person's body is able to handle and for the locals who grow up using it, it eventually because too easy to manage the effects. People with chronic illnesses put their trust in the substance, and therefore, this has led to extensive search from people all over the world.

The people from Colombia use the brew made from ayahuasca as a bonding drink. They meet at least every week to enjoy the brew together. The shaman as they call him who happens to be the village's witchdoctor joins the party every week. They take advantage of the gathering to talk about various issues affecting the community and also to share ideas on different things. It is also a learning process for the young boys who are soon going to be men. They are taught how to be men while the elders enjoy the brew. Deliberation on issues involving the community which is settled by men is made possible during this gathering. It is a brew enjoyed by the locals to mark the end of the week, and big celebrations take place and the main delicacy being the brew. It is also used as a healing brew because it is during times like this when the local who had disputes meet to start over again. Remember that it's the same plant that had been used to perform rituals to settle the disputes. Therefore when the dispute is resolved, and both parties who had the conflicts agree again, they use the brew from the ayahuasca to celebrate the newly made friendship.

Long-time friends take advantage of the brew get together to catch up with each other. They get to talk about their families, the children, and wives. Therefore the mixture can be attributed to strengthening friendship bonds. Young men who want to get married will talk to their elders about their intentions during these gatherings. The elders may also advice young men on matters of marriage during these gatherings. Young men who are also not being good in the community are given warnings during such times. This may include young men who have made young girls pregnant but refuse to take responsibility; But more importantly, without these gathering, there would be no way to pass the communities traditions. Therefore to ensure that the cultures do not waste or are not forgotten, the older men take this opportunity to teach the young men the traditions. The women are also not left behind as they get to meet, cook, and enjoy songs and dances with the others. It is also an excellent opportunity to meet the local witchdoctor for the locals because it's the only time he is not engaged with his weekly tasks. The witch doctors are usually very busy as they are involved in the preparation of the medication, the brews and also in constant standby for people needing them for treatment. People recovering from the treatment administered to them from the ayahuasca substance are taken to the gatherings for celebrations. It helps them relax and also help them forget the effects their bodies are going through. Most will be in the crowds feeling sick and physically weak, but it is an excellent time for them as they will end up forgetting the effects for a while. This is considered as a therapy for the patients. After some time it gives a person who has consumed the brew some sense of unexplainable peace.

Ayahuasca is said to give people visualization and therefore is used to help people relax. When one is relaxed, they are able to find happiness. With the many hardships in the village, many locals look for all the ways to find happiness. It helps them with their hard day's work because visualization helps them look beyond their limits. No matter how hard the tasks seem, they are able to pull through because the herbs create the perception that the work will be easy. Therefore the locals make a concoction from the herb that will help accomplish the daily tasks. The locals believe the mixture removes the laziness and also makes the more energetic so that they are able to work. Although there are experienced shamans who have the wisdom to make the mix to ensure that there is no overdose, most people continue to make the mix themselves. It is not, however very dangerous for them because with their experiences, growing up and up and watching it mix has made it easy for them. The mix is taken as an energizer but in a tiny portion lest it becomes an overdose.

It is also much used in spiritual ceremonies with the supervision of a well-experienced shaman. In some countries like Peru, it is forbidden for locals to consume the mix without the authority of the shaman. The government may not be doing so much in following this law to ensure that it is implemented. However, the shamans understand the dangers it could cause to people if they did it wrong. But the people know the risks they could potentially pose for themselves. In ceremonies, however, the shamans are always facilitating the ceremonies. This makes it the best place for anyone who will try the mix because they are usual; they are not only safe but also consuming the right mix. The shamans are trustable because they know which other medications may not go well with this mix. The locals may get the mix right, but they may not know what drugs would react negatively if they added the substance.

Since ayahuasca is said to help people travel to the other world, traditionally it is used by people who feel they want to disconnect with reality. This could be people who have gone through hard times and would want to get rid of their pains and worries. This could be effective because consumption makes someone high for not less than six hours. Imagine disconnection for six hours. This could lead to someone going through a whole self-reflection session that will help them conquer their worst fears. Not to forget that the locals think that you can connect to a greater being than yourself. Therefore this could help them connect with the greater being that will help them in getting rid of the old life. Getting disconnected erases memories of fear and pain and creates new memories.

Ayahuasca is also used as a charm traditionally. For men and women who have sexual issues, it is used to help boost their libidos. The people believe that it allows couples who are struggling with having children. This has led to the abuse of this mix as people use it even when it's for merely sexual pleasures. But for people who really need it, the shaman administers portions that help them with the problem.

People also seek the shaman to get a dose to help them get rid of witchcraft spells. It is said to protect people from being bewitched by their jealousy neighbors. Also for people who feel like things are not working out for them because they have been bewitched, the shaman always has a curative mix from ayahuasca that treats them. It is believed to treat all kinds of damaging emotions, including anger issues. Therefore when someone is going through emotions they feel they cannot handle, they seek a special mix from the shaman that helps get rid of these damaging emotions. When someone has doubts about their partner's unfaithfulness, they seek help from the shaman who administers the portion that will help figure it out. When couples are having conflicts among themselves, they are given a portion that helps them overcome the conflicts. When people are doubting loyalty in their friendships, they seek the intervention of the healers to help administer them a special portion that will help them identify their disloyal friends.

The ayahuasca has been credited for healing very strange illness for the locals. The disease that is sometimes blamed on witchcraft, it is combined with other sacred plant remedies that create a healing potion that heals the person. The thing with ayahuasca is that the locals strongly believe it is a spirit plant and that the spirits work through the healers to administer healing. Therefore even before consumption of the portion, the ill people seek a way to appease the spirits.

The elders use the ayahuasca plant during rituals to help catch thieves. When there are unexplainable calamities like thieves who have not been caught, the rituals will help them in establishing who the thieves are. It is also used by the healers to communicate useful information that has been communicated to them by the spirits. It is also used to explain mysteries happening in the community because it could be a way for the spirits communicating their displeasure with the people. When it is found that the spirits are unhappy, they use the same plant to perform rituals that will appeal to the spirits for forgiveness. It is mainly used to link the people to the spirits. The communication is both ways when the spirits need to pass information; they pass it through the healers. When people want advice for the people from the spirits, they perform rituals. The ayahuasca is, therefore, a very sacred plant traditionally for its people.

CHAPTER 7
Different Uses For Ayahuasca And Why One Would Choose A Certain Use

Ayahuasca has different uses. The uses depend on who is using it; the shaman, members of Brazilian churches, indigenous people of the Amazon, dark shamans or some ritualists. Here are the different uses of this mysterious plant.

Shamanic/Traditional Use

Ayahuasca is used widely is shamanism. Different tribes from Bolivia to Colombia use it. Shamans use ayahuasca and other range of plants as spiritual entities. These plants are believed to have character and consciousness. Shamans are like doctors, and their knowledge is passed down from generation to generation. Shamans use it for different uses:

1) **Healing use**

Ayahuasca can heal all kinds of illnesses. During the weekly ayahuasca ceremony organized by the shaman, there are the brew and plant spirits. The combination of these three things brings healing to participants. The participants drink an ounce of the brew which is bitter and unpleasant to everyone. During this ceremony, the shaman and the participants sit in the dark for some time to allow the effect of ayahuasca to be felt. In some cases, the shaman sings and makes some whistling sound immediately the participants drink the brew.

In around an hour after drinking the brew, the participants start to get visions. The visions keep on increasing, and at the same time, the shaman continues to sing the "icaros". Many people have been healed from mental problems, emotional disorders, physical problems and many cases of rising from the dead. There are also a great number of people who have testified on receiving healing from their addictions.

2) **Sorcery use**

Using ayahuasca for sorcery is common among the Amazon Shamanism. The shamans are lured into using their knowledge to harm others. A true shaman should have control, and lack of it might lead him/her to sorcery. In shamanism, some shamans are not beneficial to their participants. Some shamans use their powers to steal power from their clients. Some use sorcery to attract more customers and make them return. They also use their power for seduction. Shamanic powers indeed heal but at a price. Some shamans will claim to be beneficial to their clients, but the results are always devastating. Some clients get mental problems, and some even die. Some clients also go to some dark shamans to get sorcery services like to have powers to seduce their dream partners.

3) Initiation use

Shamans are initiated through the use of ayahuasca. The shaman influences his initiate, and they both meet with a common purpose and respect. This experience depends on the initiate's reaction, and it can be pleasant or unpleasant. The initiation ceremony is premeditated to evade madness. The shaman is accountable for the initiate's spiritual and mental health. They do this practice with respect and a lot of trusts. During this process, there is drumming used as a warm-up. In an initiation ceremony, there is only one initiate at a time due to the dangerous nature of the process. Ayahuasca is a great teacher to aspiring shamans. The initiates take the plant with the addition of some diets over some time.

4) Contacting spirits

Many shamans get permission from spirits to learn on how to use different plants for healing. Shamans use 'icaros' also understood as medicine songs to summon spirits. The spirit intended to be summoned the shaman its song before being summoned. They use ayahuasca and some totemic items to get special powers. The spirits are invoked to officiate the ceremony or to only be in the presence. In some cases, the spirits take over the shaman's body and lead the ceremony. In such a case, the shaman gets the ability to transverse other dimensions and gets visions and information.

Hybrid Rituals

Different groups developed their ayahuasca ceremonies after being inspired by the indigenous ceremonies. Some groups use new-age shamanic techniques or merge with the ayahuasca drink. The hybrid rituals are being performed in the Western world and Latin-America. They invoke the spirits to ask for guidance and protection. They also use power animals and plants. Just like in traditional use, participants use different tactics like dancing, drumming, and breathing exercises. There is a presence of some ritual tools like candles, incense, flowers and Buddha or saints. Sometimes there is music; live musicians or recorded music.

The participants gather in a circle around a fire outside or sometimes in a room. They don't sit as it happens in churches, but they lay down on separate mattresses. The biggest part of the ritual is spent in silence to allow participants to travel inwards, but some parts involve singing. They share experiences using a piece of the ayahuasca vine. This ritual is led by a shaman or sometimes people with ayahuasca experiences.

Therapeutic Use

Other than the shamans, therapists got curious about the miracle brew. Scientific studies have been conducted to find out the effects of ayahuasca as a medicine. Most studies concluded that consumption of ayahuasca had no psychological or physical effects and did not show signs of addiction. Here are different ways ayahuasca is used as a therapy.

1. Treating severe depression

Some people who have taken ayahuasca before have said they felt at peace with God, universe and themselves. In today's scientific studies, people who took ayahuasca had the acute effects of it for about four hours. The acute effects included vomiting, dream-like visions, and introspection. The scientific studies have shown that 64% of the patients get healed from depression by using ayahuasca.

2. Treating addictions

We are all aware of how ayahuasca was used in healing processes for thousands of years by the shamans. Despite them using it for a long time, it was only recently that it got recognition from the public. Its treatment of drug addiction was only explored recently in Western science. Gabe Mate, an expert believes that ayahuasca has the power to treat the psychological pain faced by people struggling with addictions. A study on a few people who took ayahuasca showed the following results:

- Their well-being improved.
- They reduced their intake of tobacco, cocaine, and alcohol.
- They did not have harmful side effects after taking ayahuasca.

In the long-run, it is a good addiction treatment because, after two years of the initial study, the individuals reported positive results including:

- They had abstained from drugs for two years or reduced their intake.
- They understood the cause of their addictions.
- Their problem-solving behavior improved.
- More than 50% of them reduced their cravings after ingesting ayahuasca.

How does ayahuasca treat addiction?

- No talking involved- Ayahuasca gives a non-verbal treatment unlike the therapies of today. Most people have a problem in expressing their feelings and thoughts and especially to strangers. Lack of talking enables the addicts to use their other senses to facilitate spiritual and psychological treatment.
- Improves mental health- Ayahuasca therapy has been linked to a decrease in the symptoms of anxiety and depression.
- It heals- People with past experiences from ayahuasca ceremonies have reported healing from some trauma and

past distress. It has been made possible by reflecting and having an increased insight on their past experiences. Ayahuasca also helps people to open up to the shamans without problems.
- It provides a different mindset- The hallucinogenic experiences caused by ingesting ayahuasca make people change their mindset. Ayahuasca induces confidence, pride and empowerment feelings. It also makes you connected to the environment, self and other people as well as being mindful.
- It can assist in enabling biology- Its therapy improves serotonin activity. It regulates a person's frame of mind and reduces urges of substances in addicts.

3. Preventing suicides

Ayahuasca gives you the ability to question your mind. You are gifted with an ability to question things that you might have known as the gospel truth all your life. You dig into the root of your problem. You not only remember the cause may be childhood trauma, but you feel the feelings experienced during the trauma. Many people have testified that ayahuasca gave them purpose in life thus preventing them from committing suicide.

4. Pain

Many people have been healed of their physical pains after taking ayahuasca. To some, it did not happen after the first day of ingestion, but to most, it was instant. They reported that during the ceremony they felt as if the drink was scanning their bodies to find areas that needed help. Most people with multiple causes' conditions like backaches sleep disorders and fatigue benefit greatly from ayahuasca.

5. Anxiety

After the first process of ayahuasca, you are given a window for change about 2 to 4 weeks. During this window, you feel happy and relaxed, and this gives you a chance to change your life. Ayahuasca gives you the ability to know what happened in your journey and helps you to work it out through changes. Processing your journey is not an easy task as it involves getting metaphoric images in your mind that you are supposed to deduce their meaning. Ayahuasca gives you peace.

6. Grief therapy

Death of the people who are close to us and those that we love dearly is not a good thing to experience. People use ayahuasca to lower their levels of grief. Ayahuasca gives you the ability to connect with the person that you lost. You will not see the person, but you feel them and get an opportunity to tie loose ends, which brings you closure.

Personal Growth

Ayahuasca has received an increase in its use as a spiritual and enlightenment tool in recent years. Many people who have sought help on personal growth have given back positive results. They say that they experience compassion for people around them and a connection to them. Some said they received spiritual awakening that gave them a stable shift on their perception of others and their surroundings. Ayahuasca gives its users the ability to connect with nature.

Many entrepreneurs are also seeking ayahuasca's help, and many people of any influence in the world are using ayahuasca. Its use gives you a connection with your clients. Some people who have had anger issues claimed that they disappeared after using Ayahuasca. Some people in the tech industry use ayahuasca to get creative. They claim that ayahuasca helps them to dive into their subconscious. It does not give an instant reaction, but it helps in the spirituality and creativity process. Most experts in the tech industry say they experienced emotional freedom and new creativity and as a result, they get growth in their minds and financially.

Reasons for Choosing Certain Use of Ayahuasca

We have discussed four uses of ayahuasca above. Now, let us find out why people choose the above uses for ayahuasca.

Shamanic/Traditional Use

To get physical healing

Many people suffering from chronic illnesses have found healing after using ayahuasca. Every individual is different; some take long while others take shorter periods. The shamans usually determine this. Some people have also sought ayahuasca to be healed from diabetes.

To cause harm

Some shamans use ayahuasca in their sorcery. There is nothing good found in sorcery other than to harm others. Dark shaman's use it to steal powers from their clients. Participants visit the shamans to receive sorcery to do several things; to attract customers to their business, to win in seducing someone else, to harm a competitor, etc. Sorcery is used to make people do something they would not do without being pushed by dark forces. Getting powers to seduce someone who would initially not go out with you is wrong, and it might cause harm in the future to that person. Some shamans even use their powers to kill others.

Completion of the ritual

Shamans use the ayahuasca plant to invoke spirits to the ayahuasca ceremony. Without the presence of the spirits in the ceremony, the ceremony would be incomplete. The presence of the spirits gives the participants the ability to travel to the spiritual world in the form of hallucinations.

Continuation of the shaman's practices

Shaman's use ayahuasca in the initiation process of a new shaman. They take the plant together with a specific diet, and this completes the initiation process. Ayahuasca gives hope for the future shaman practices. The ayahuasca practices are passed from generations to generations through intense teachings, the connection of the spirits and mind.

Hybrid Rituals

To tap into a superior sense of wonder and mystery

Ayahuasca guides you through mystery and pure magic. You experience extreme beauty as you've never seen. You feel so much joy within you; too much for your body to accommodate till you weep like a child.

To ask for protection and guidance

We mentioned before of the new age shamanic groups that use ayahuasca drink to invoke spirits. They request for the spirit's protection from harm and guidance in life. Some shamans need protection from the dark shamans who use their power for wrong reasons and to cause harm. During ayahuasca ceremony, the spirits appear to the shamans or sometimes merge with his body to relay messages of assured protection and messages on how to live life.

Therapeutic Use

To find answers

Many people seek ayahuasca's treatment to find answers to essential questions about life, including path, relationships, and career. Some want answers to specific questions while others give their intentions and they are given answers.

To cleanse the body

Ayahuasca cleanses the body from all toxins like drugs and substance in the system as well as emotional pains in our systems. Some participants purge, sweats and other vomit. These processes enable them to release dark mass-energy from the body. Some people purge throughout the ceremony, but in their bucket, there is no vomit. Others purge through moaning, laughing, coughing, and crying. Those are emotional purges.

To improve their mental health

Ayahuasca is believed to heal sources of trauma like childhood abuse. These traumas cause anxiety or PTSD. It does so by uncovering the cause, and a person purges those feelings out permanently. It is not a comfortable thing to experience, but it is effective and good medicine.

Regain your power

Some of us may have lost their powers because of the different traumas we have experienced. After one or several ceremonies, you feel the power come running back to you. You feel a little of yourself return and gain more power and authority. You feel as if you are being broken down and then integrated into something new. The result is freedom; freedom from all the pains and trauma that you've hidden deep in your feelings for a long period.

To beat addiction

As we learned in the therapeutic use of ayahuasca, it cleanses one's system from all addictions, and there is never a relapse. Many people have used ayahuasca to overcome alcohol and drug addiction.

To find your purpose in life

In ayahuasca's therapeutic use, we mentioned that it prevents people from committing suicide. People with strong emotions and thoughts of committing suicide have changed their mind after taking ayahuasca. Ayahuasca takes you to a higher dimension where you are broken into pieces then integrated back as one whole piece. In the spiritual realm, you get to know what your purpose in life is. Some people receive guidance on their careers while others are given their purpose.

Personal Growth

Some people seek the use of ayahuasca for their personal growth. Personal growth is hindered by many things; some of them our past issues that keep cropping in our present lives. You can never walk for long with baggage on your back. Our past traumatic experiences are our baggage. Let us look at the reasons people use ayahuasca for personal growth.

Emotional healing

Ayahuasca is used to heal the body as well as the mind. After taking a dose or two of ayahuasca, you will start feeling your past emotions. You face emotions that you've been hiding for a long time caused by traumatic events. It will be a difficult procedure, but you are supposed to face them bravely and handle them for good. Your emotional burden reduces. Isn't it a fast way to healing than the long hours of therapy required to heal emotionally? With a clear soul and a happy self, that is the first step towards personal growth.

1. Spiritual progression

You will get a glimpse of the spiritual world. You will feel an illumination as you break away from the medium. You will see and feel things you've never experienced before. It will give you a good understanding of reality.

2. Finding purpose

There are some things we all feel a great push to do them, but we get scared too. Did you know that ayahuasca is called the little death? It is because when you take it, your body and mind break away from your consciousness. This feeling is more like death, and it reminds you to search for your purpose. You get a clear picture of your purpose just as you always wanted.

3. Happiness

Ayahuasca gives you happiness. You experience true happiness. All the emotional pain in our systems gets cleaned, and all the broken part become whole again. True happiness is a seed for personal growth. If you are truly happy you attract people around you, and everyone wants to be associated with you. People are assets, and they should be treasured. Happiness is a stepping stone for personal growth.

4. Tap your creativity

Artists like painters, musicians or designers need to showcase their inspirations via their respective means. They have been blessed with access to something deep and mystifying. Highly creative people have no problem with parading themselves out there and showcasing what lies internally and beyond. Sometimes these people luck inspiration. Using ayahuasca bring changes to their consciousness. They get the freedom to experience without problems and self-judgment. They get their creativity back, and they get back to business. To these kinds of people, without creativity, they are at a disadvantage and can easily lose themselves in its loss.

CHAPTER 8
The Science Behind Ayahuasca

Ayahuasca is one of the many plants that is being used by the indigenous people. It is a beverage that is known to benefit the soul as well as the body of a person. The shamans are the people known to prepare and administer the brew. You cannot make the plant tea on yourself since it requires an expert to guide you in doing that. They apply it as a way to guide the people through visual as well as auditory hallucinations. As the years go by, the brew is becoming popular in other parts of the world. It has spread because people have realized that it is an excellent remedy for treating anxiety and depression.

The mixture contains some mysterious natural compounds that will help numerous ways when you consume. It is a combination of two plants which is contrary to what most people think. The plant cannot do by itself, and it depends on other ingredients to be effective. The combination of Psychotria Viridis leaves, and Banisteriopsis caapi vines are what makes up the Ayahuasca component. None of the element can have the hallucinogenic power without the involvement of the other. The remedy is known to have DMT which is a psychoactive compound. It also contains a chemical called monoamine oxidase inhibitors. It helps in blocking the enzymes in your body that are responsible for the breaking down of DMT before it gets to your brain. DMT then gets to interact with some receptors in your mind and elevates your mood-enhancing your emotional wellbeing. That makes it a powerful ingredient to treat some psychological disorders through some neurobiological mechanisms that are behind the therapeutic effect.

The vines of the ayahuasca are the ones responsible for inhibiting the DMT enzymes from their normal functioning. The catalyst then enters the bloodstream and crosses a particular blood barrier in the brain, and that is where it all begins. The brew will start affecting you thirty minutes after you take it. You will have hallucinations after one hour, and the drug will wear off after six hours. The exciting thing is that when you are on this brew, you will know that you are having hallucinations and you will be alert. It is contrary to the illusions that you can experience when you take some other drugs.

When you are under the influence of this brew, the hallucinations that you have are different. You will hear sounds and not voices, and for that, there is some music playing when people are on an ayahuasca retreat. It will make you be at ease with your thoughts, and you will embrace your current situation without much fighting back. When you take this remedy, you will not get high, but instead, you will have the chance to reconcile with your past experiences as well as emotions. That will help you to find the inner peace that is most crucial to your daily life. That means that there are unique things that happen in your brain to have such an effect.

Ayahuasca has high content that can be of great help in fighting cancer. Using this drug will increase some characters that associate with mindfulness. It is one of the approaches that are put in use to help fight depression as well as anxiety. If you have a case of PTSD or grief, this will be an excellent thing for you to try and have your healthy life back. The magic remedy provides compelling evidence that it has some therapeutic powers. That stimulates the creation of neurons in the brain, and hence it serves as an of regenerating brain cells that could be in one way or the other damaged.

Good enough, science is backing up all the medical benefits that are known to stem from this magical brew. The plant medicine needs handling with a lot of respect because of the danger that is attached to it. When you decide to go for the mixture, you need to change your diet as well as any prescription that you may be having. Some medications never go hand in hand with this drug and the need for you to suspend them. You need to clean your system of any toxins that may have accumulated with time. You need to take a diet called twenty days before you start the journey with the brew. It will prepare you and boost your ability to receive the benefits of the herb. If you do not take the diet, you will get it hard to handle the drug effects. And for you to get a high consciousness state, the overall toxicity levels need to be lower. That is the reason that you need to be dangerous in taking the diet. The more you will discipline, the more the medicine is likely to be effective. If you do not practice honesty with the prescription, you might find things getting sour.

The herb has a notable medical benefit when administered in the right way. You are likely to have experiences that are frightening when you use the drug despite the fact that it is a promising treatment. For that, you need to make sure that you are in the company of people who can take good care of you. Do not take the experience lightly ad, so you need to before you partake the brew. You can get into a vulnerable situation, and in some cases, the effect may be intense. When you finally use the herb, you need to have its full information. When done in the right way, you can have a beautiful journey. When you mix with some foods, it can even lead to death, and so you need to take caution.

As outlined earlier, Ayahuasca refers to a psychedelic brew that was traditionally used by Amerindians. It is a brew that was made from leaves of Psychotria Viridis shrub along the stalk of Banisteriopsis caapi vine as well as other plants that are essential ingredients. It is worth noting that the drink was used for religious and spiritual purposes by the ancient Amazonian tribes. Nowadays, the brew is used as a sacred beverage by most of the religious communities in North America as well as Brazil. Traditionally the mixture was prepared by an experienced healer who was the leader of major Ayahuasca ceremonies. Boiling leaves in water made the mixture. The psychoactive drink was made from the barks of Banisteriopsis. The plant is rich in beta-Caroline harmala alkaloids with N, N- dimethyltryptamine. The brew also contains harmine and harmaline alkaloids that are oxidase inhibitors. The mixture was initially utilized by Amazonian shamans in ritual ceremonies as well as folk healers for several reasons. It is worth noting that the reason for the growing interest as well as the increasing usage of Ayahuasca was due to the safety as well as the behavioral effects, let alone the clinical use of the brew. In other words, the mixture had several medical importances hence a need to be utilized in various ceremonies. The combination was known to be a potential treatment in addictions, depressions as well as anxiety. Thus, the usage of Ayahuasca dates back to the aboriginal inhabitants of the Amazon basin. It was utilized as an indigenous shaman for communicating with the magical experiences, rites of passage as well in healing rituals. In other words, it is the brew thought to be connecting the living with the dead. The mixture was poured to the ground before any ceremony as a means of connecting the life with the dead it was the perfect drink for doing so.

Psychological Effects

The experience of Ayahuasca begins approximately 40 minutes after ingestion. The effect of the brew peak between the 60th and the 120th minute. The subjective effects in most cases fade after a period of about 4 hours.it is worth noting that the impact of the drug isn't so intense such that the hallucinations don't last for long. In most cases, the victim doesn't lose consciousness, but they may experience an alteration in it. However, in fact of an injection, the individuals tend to experience extended loss of knowledge within a short period. Some of the most common psychological effects that are reported after Ayahuasca ingestion include a powerful feeling of self-confidence as well as a new perspective over all aspects of life. In other words, the chemical component in the blew affect the mindset of an individual where it causes an alteration that might be chronic if the blew has overdosed. However, if small and adequate measures are taken, the blew plays a critical role in altering the mindset of an individual positively. In most after ingesting Ayahuasca, 30 minutes later, most subjects' notes a change in the perception and shaking might be noted. The victim is reported to be more vulnerable and is easily influenced. Shortly after, most of the participants experience some sense of confusions, fear as well as paranoia.
In most cases, the victim's defensive mechanism is diminished, and the participants tend to experience a shift in the expansive state and may peak in vomiting and feeling nausea. Other participants complain of feeling a transcendental experience in the spiritual world. Most of them

encounter plant and animal spirit and may even contact a higher sense. There are reports of feeling united with the universe, and there are profound peace and ecstasy to those who allow the spirits to carry them. In most cases, the participant's feels more united with the dead and tend to experience some sense of timelessness, and at times the timing may speed or slow depending on the onset of the feeling. However, as victims have all these sensations, they remain aware of their surroundings and can even speak as if they are sober.

In most cases, the victims feel attached to the spirits and tend to receive useful lessons from the spirit teachers. In other words, one may feel the aspect of the spirit world being drained and get connected more to the spirit world. There are cases where the visual element tends to fade, and one feels as if they don't want to remain in the physical world again.

Several studies have been carried out to identify the hallucinogenic properties of Ayahuasca. It has been determined that Ayahuasca has several effects that cause the increased art of hallucinations. Some of these effects include the somatic impact that affects the way a person feels. The results might feel emotionally disoriented and lose focus in a way. The other consequence is on volition, where the willful desire to interact might be altered. The victim may also have some difficulties in cognition as well as their perception. The intensity of doing things might increase depending on what they feel. Some victims have been reported to experience increased activation as well as the art of euphoria at all times. The aspect has been linked to the fact that, after ingestion, the concentration of Ayahuasca increases in the plasma.

In most cases, if the individual had consumed Ayahuasca earlier, the effect tends to be intense. The aspect is linked to the fact that the minds tend to recap the feeling, and as the concentration increases due to absorption, the effects tend to be more vivid. It is worth noting that the dosage used dictates whether the period over which these effects reach. In most cases, a dosage of more than 0.85g of Ayahuasca content tends to be more than enough to strike an onset of the impact. However, high doses are required if the victim had used Ayahuasca in the past. The aspect is due to the fact that the body might have been used to the dosage hence a need to add on the hallucinogen.

Long-term Psychological Effects

There have been studies carried out to investigate the effects of continuous use of Ayahuasca. It is worth noting that there are people who live in churches which use Ayahuasca daily. In most cases, the leaders of the rituals tend to consume Ayahuasca quit often. However, some haven't tasted it. In the study, they were used as the control test. It was noted that the addiction such as the use of alcohol and sickness such as depression and anxiety tend to be remitted once someone gets used to Ayahuasca. In most, it was challenging to identify whether the effects on the kids on adolescent was due to Ayahuasca or the religious teachings. The aspect is linked to the fact that there are tremendous effects that occur to a person who receives such instructions. It is worth noting that most victims of Ayahuasca are more attached to the spirit and the teaching they receive in the spiritual world changes their perception. In the same way, the kids who are under such instructions in the physical world may have similar effects.

The Brain structure of Ayahuasca

It is worth noting that Ayahuasca has a more significant impact on the mindset of an individual. In other words, the brew tends to alter the brain areas hence the hallucination. In most cases, the higher the concentration, the higher the effect hence notifiable changes. In most cases, the brain is altered, and a victim tends to overdo things. For instances, there are reports of re-examination of issues, and people tend to experience the art of re-experiencing negative memories and developing problems with emotional distress. In other words, the rate of amygdala tends to increase, and the painting brings back the full memory of adverse situations. There are cases where the utilization rate of Ayahuasca comes with an effect on the art of consciousness and may increase the self-understanding of an individual. The victim might have an altered perception and might develop some difficulties in recognizing issues. For instance, there cases where the religious leaders who are frequent users of Ayahuasca tend to forget their roles, and at times they may overdo them. The aspect is linked to the fact that most of the time, they feel attached to the spirit world and handles more asserted or connived to the things of the spirit. Most of them may lose control over the art of processing information. In other words, there are cases where victims lose the art of listening and speaking. In other words, they may develop some issues when it comes to speaking or instead of listening to what one may have to say. Most of the site issues to do with the spirit and users who are under the influence of Ayahuasca you may never understand their feelings as well. However, most of the Ayahuasca changes that occur in the brain affect the emotions of an individual. In other words, the changes that re reduced are mainly focused on the mind. In most cases, when the dosage is done in the right way, the changes occur in the rots way, and the victim brings a positive difference. For instance, there are cases where an individual has changed from addiction as well as some recovering from anxiety as well as other mental disorders. The aspect is linked to the fact that Ayahuasca mostly reaches the brain and alters the thinking of an individual.

Safety and Adverse Effects

The low dosage of Ayahuasca doesn't have any adverse effect on the brain of a victim. However, the art of over-dependent tends to increase the rate at which changes occurs within an individual. In most cases, hallucinations tend to be intense in the case of over-dependence. However, one of the adverse effects of low dosages is that it causes one to crave more and in the long run, fall into addiction.

In most cases, Ayahuasca tends to suppress the sensory aspect that increases the art of hallucination.

In most cases, there are significant changes in the sensory element such that increased delusion may cause the art of vomiting. The aspect is due to the fact that increased serotonin stimulates the vagus nerve and may cause diarrhea. There are cases where the blood pressure and the heart rate may also increase.

Under normal conditions, the bodies destroy any form of DMT in the systems. There is a monoamine oxidase in the order that helps in destroying these DMT. However, Ayahuasca contains a Monoamine oxidase inhibitor that prevents the escape of DMT as well as the alteration of consciousness. It is worth noting that most of the depression, as well as anxiety disorders, tend to be caused by the failure of reabsorption of serotonin. When DMT is maintained, it binds in the same sights with serotonin. Thus its level in the system remains the same; hence, the recovery from any form of depression as well as anxiety. In other words, the DMT bids in the sites that serotonin should bind. The aspect is critical in the sense that it serotonin is left unbound in the system. Its continuous re-absorption helps individuals recover from mental conditions. It is worth noting that most of this mental condition affects the state of mind. A negative perception as well anxiety may heighten the situation, and the person may remain in this condition forever. However, with Ayahuasca, more serotonin is re-absorbed is achieved. The aspect is critical in the sense that it enhances the restructuring of the brain hence the fast recovery.

The Ayahuasca effect is also critical in aiding brain recovery as well as the processing of information. In other words, the brain areas where dopamine and serotonin receptors are less, the GABA in the Ayahuasca cause one to feel the uninhabited effect. Such a result is critical in the sense that it opens one's mind, and there are chances of increase in terms of one's productivity. In other words, the Ayahuasca effect causes the mind's receptors to be more productive, and more serotonin is reabsorption. The art of re-absorption enhances a cooling effect that is critical in weaving after a recovering of anxiety.

CHAPTER 9
Effects Of Ayahuasca On Body, Brain, And Consciousness

Ayahuasca is a tea plant with the origin of South America and is used by indigenous people for religion purposes. It is known to contain therapeutic potential when it comes to treating mental disorders. It is as well crucial in enhancing capacities related to mindfulness. It has sub-acute as well as long-term improvement to the users when it comes to cognitive thinking. It helps someone who has negative thoughts in that they will be in a position to accept and not self-judge in any way. They will not react to unusual environments or situations when they. The drug has a mysterious way of dealing with the overall healing. It can either be physical, emotional, spiritual, as well as mental healing bearing in mind that they have a unique way that they connect. It is an excellent remedy that will bring to an end even some of the terminal illnesses. It will help you to overcome post-traumatic stress disorder, and you will be in a position to regulate the emotions that come along. It is known to work better for PTSD patients than when they go for therapies.

Ayahuasca is an excellent remedy to increase the levels of creativity and raises divergent thinking and bringing down convergent thinking. When you use this tea plant, you will be psychologically flexible, and you will cope in a fast way. It is known to be an excellent depressant when taken by someone who is fighting depression. The way ayahuasca functions and the effects it will have will vary from one person to the other. They have a very long as well as powerful experience once used. It will change your life-transforming you to a different person with new spirits as well as energy. Though people h, this drug will help you overcome any doubt in you. They will no longer be an obstacle in your life. Numerous effects come with the use of the drug. They include and not limited to;

Makes the Unconscious Conscious

It is made possible because of the raised levels of dopamine that makes the pleasure centers to be more active. It will make your personal experiences integrated. The integration, as well as the processing, will go forward, and you are likely to experience full emotions. The experience will not come to a stop by the things that were making the process to stop. The prefrontal cortex will not have the ability to limit the decisions that you will make since GABA will come. There will be no bodily feedback, as well. There will be no chances that the trauma will re-visit you, and the cycle of avoidance will be interrupted. Your ability to judge as well as to repress the fear in one way or the other controlled. You will witness it as one of the direct results. The neural activities will increase in some areas of the brain that are responsible for integrating the memory and experience emotions. You will experience a high level of consciousness. You cannot solve a problem if it is in the same consciousness level that it has come. Some of the issues that we experience roots from lack of consciousness. When your levels of consciousness go up, you will have no one to direct you on the way to live your life. You will find it automatic that you can do things in the right direction and in a natural way. You will change and be someone else better than the person you was before.

Improves Eating Behaviors and Helps Fight Drug Addiction

When you drink this drug, you will feel more aware of your mind as well as body. If you have a case of drug cravings, the tea plank will help subdue such urges. The drug will as well help you to overcome your eating disorders and many more diseases that you might be suffering from. It will boost your urge to take food that you were taking before. It can as well treat some mental health disorders due to a psychoactive feeling that comes as a result of receptors having an activation. If you have cases of trauma, you will be in a position to understand that more and the exact thing that triggers you into it. Hence you can constructively deal with your issues. It is an excellent remedy for fighting drug addiction. For alcohol abusers, it can be of great help in controlling the way they consume. They are chemically reconstructed in the brain receptors, and it confronts the problem that made to indulge in drug abuse. A drug addict will then reduce the amount of drug they take since the cravings will go to a lower level.

It Restores Self-Esteem

When you use ayahuasca, you will have an energy boost, and you will have your levels of self-esteem go up. When you have self-confidence, you will have the courage to face a lot in your life. You can fight the issues that stress you, and for that, you will prevent depression from hitting you. In cases where one is already suffering from depression, it will give you an idea of how you resolve your past trauma and forge ahead with life. The benefits are in association with the soul, and it will ease the hardship that you can suffer because of depression. You will understand yourself, and you can implement a meaningful as well as lasting improvement in your life. You will have that chance to ask yourself who the exact person you are and how to continue with your life. You can live forever trying to find out the correct person you are, but when you take this remedy, you will find it easy. The things that you are not in a position to know when you are in a conscious state, you will see when you are under the influence of this drug. You will go deeper into your thoughts, and you will have a revelation of who you are. You will do away with all the things that distract you from self-realization and also the way you judge yourself will automatically change.

Help you Find your Purpose in Life

Finding the meaning of one's life is the main reason why people will attend the ayahuasca retreats. When you take in the drug, you will find a new direction that you will take in your life to achieve the best. You will start the awakening process, and you will know what exactly to do with your life. You will have an idea of who you are in the spiritual world, and you will have a reason to continue fighting until you make it. You will know the purpose of your life, and you will not live blindly after that. You are likely to make a significant change after you take this magical drink. You will venture into the things that are fulfilling to you, and that will make you live a life of joy and a healthier one. You will have a deep connection to nature, and that will change your lifestyle and also the perception of how you view the world. The experience is known to have a long-term effect meaning that it will not disappear when the drug wears off. When you take this drug away from your usual environment, it will be vital to help you disconnect. You will have a good time away from all the distractions, and in that way, you can have a peaceful moment to determine the exact purpose of your life. You should consider going to the jungle since it has a natural way of making you feel deeper as well as closer to the natural world.

It Will Help You Appreciate Life

One of the most significant benefits that you can get from this drug is being able to understand life in a more profound way. You will understand what life has given you and the things that are about to offer you. You will appreciate nature, your life as well as the universe knowing how the connection it has and the role it plays in your life. That overwhelming feeling of being grateful to the people around you will be the result when you take the remedy. When you are thankful for all the things that life has given you, you will have a happy life. A healthier life will make you establish a good relationship with the things that you come on your way, and you will live a harmonious life.

It Helps Clean Your Body

Ayahuasca is popularly known for its ability to cleanse the body. It helps to detoxify the gallbladder, liver as well as the blood. It will reduce the risks of you getting diabetes and cancer. It slows down the process of natural medicine and increases its effectiveness in inhibiting the growth of cells that are associated with the disease. It helps in stimulating and creating of neurons in your brain, decreasing the effects of the emissions that can be made by Alzheimer. The illnesses that come along with the faults in the flow of blood w once you take the tea plant. It will be for you to give it a try and see how great it will work for you. It not only provokes hallucinations but also it is known for inducing purging. It is a pleasant experience, but it will help to detoxify the body. It will clean the guts and responsible for removing all the parasites and microorganisms that are lurking. The presence of parasites in your body will do you more harm than good. The parasites will damage the metabolic system and cause you diseases that may cause you to be bedridden. The detoxification is physical as well as chemical. When you take this ingredient, you will eliminate the harmful microorganisms, and you can enjoy your good health. It leaves the digestive tract with no infections making it smooth for digestion to take place. The tea as well contains a chemical that will kill the parasites that are in your body system.

Contains an Anti-Depression Effect

The drug serves as an excellent remedy for your health in terms of emotions. The brain part in charge of processing emotions, as well as motivations, will be stimulated hence the reduction of depression and the feeling of anxiety. When you take ayahuasca tea, you are likely to vomit. It is not a pleasant experience since it comes along with some benefits. It is responsible for regulating your mood by stimulating the flow of blood to your brain. The DMT is a compound found in the substance and it the one that activates receptors which are in charge of improving your mood. Depression is a great inconvenience, and it will disrupt your life, making it hard for you to have a healthy life. It will keep you away from doing the things that you love most. Depression as well threatens your life, and taking this drug will help to get back to your healthy life.

It Helps One to Stop Abusing Substances

The tea plant is known to contain hallucinogenic properties. Even though it is associated with one being high, it will make you to remain calm as well as composed in the entire process. If you want to win-off from particular substances, the tea will be an excellent idea for you to try out. When you take a moderate amount, you will have amazing results. It comes along with psychological as well as spiritual benefits and reduces the craving that you may have for substances. It will help you be creative and be in a position to recover from your addiction positively. It will change your behavior, and you will have a reduction in the desire to take your substance of choice often.

Reduces the Risk Associated With Cancer

Cancer is the number one disease that is leading to massive deaths across the entire globe. An excellent remedy that will help people to fight cancer will be an addition for the people. Ayahuasca is an excellent remedy when it comes to reducing the risk of getting cancer. It will be a great way to prevent disease but will not cure cancer that is already in existence. It will reduce the number of cells that cause cancer in your body. That is made possible by the fact that the number of white blood cells multiplying. That will allow the body to combat the cells in a more natural way. It is an excellent remedy that can be used to treat cancer.

Despite the long list of the benefits of the plant, it also has some adverse effects. They include;

Though it is an excellent remedy for depression, it does not change the personality

It is useful in treating depression and more vital when it comes to lifting it. Nevertheless, when the lifting comes in, the underlying character does not change. If you use the drug because of some personality issues besides depression or trauma, the problems will not come to an end. Depression goes, but you will remain with the other aspects to battle. The grief you had will be replaced with the feeling of anger. That anger might stem from the traumatic abuses that you went through before you got into depression. Though the drug will give you the ability as well as the opportunity to work things out, it will not necessarily do them for you.

Your Mood will be Worse than Before

When you use the plant, you will be re-visited by some of the traumatic events that happened some time back. You will have fear, paranoia as well as the feeling of being emotionally hurt. When any user experiences such an effect, they will choose to drop the drug and sort for an alternative. They are likely to experience bad trips. Your general mood will change, and you can feel confused and your way of thinking disorganized. In some instances, it will make someone be emotionally traumatized.

Visual as well as Auditory Hallucinations

The tea plant is known to have disturbances as well as changes in the way one will see the things that surround them. They will see as if the things that are within the same environment have intensified in terms of color. When you use this drug, you will experience changes in time experience. You will either see as if time is moving on quickly or slower than it usually does. The hallucinations that you will experience will have a theme which in most cases, it turns out to be of the ancient civilization, futuristic or it either personifies the nature itself. The closed-eye hallucinations are more profound, and the user will go to a different world of their own. That does not exclude open-eyed hallucinations that are also part of what one is likely to experience. Many of the users will have experiences that are out of the body. You will feel in your intense body vibrations that are from the physical surroundings. You will see and hear things that are not real and do not exist.

Problem on Vision

When you are under the influence of this tree plant, you are likely to have a double image. Your eyes will experience troubles when it comes to focusing on things. The pupils will dilate, which is not the case when one is healthy. You will not be in a position to control your eye movement, and it will be rapid.

Health Disorders

You will have several health disorders when you use ayahuasca. You will have cases of increased bowel movements. When the drug is for ceremonial purposes, the one who is administering will give you instructions. That will help you to mitigate the effect that leads to increased bowel movements. When you take a high dose, your blood pressure is likely to shoot as well as your heart rate, and there can be causes of chest pain. You may have symptoms that are related to fever, and you will be dizzy at times. It can make you have nausea and in extreme cases can cause you to vomit from time to time. The effect will escalate when you have instances of a heart disorder, and it will bum uh vital that you do not try or think of taking this drug. There have been death cases that have after the use of this tea plant. It can be risky and at times, yield good fruits depending on the response you will give as well as the fate. So, you need to take care and keep your health as well as legalities before anything else.

The tea is bitter, and it can off-keep you which most people do not find it pleasing. For you to take it, you need to be having strong shock absorbers and a lot of mental strength for it to go down. It has side effects when it comes to small babies, and for that, pregnant and breastfeeding mothers should not take the concoction. The adverse effects will negatively influence the health of your baby. You must accept the dose, consult your doctor on the right dosage to make so that you can know the amount to consume. The healing that comes with this substance is long-term. You need to be sure that you do not abuse it for its long-term effects. When you have to take in large quantities, make sure it will be safe for you. You must have health conditions so that you can take this remedy. You will be in a position to take the world differently and make you more creative. It will get you out of the way you usually think and give you a chance to explore new ideas. Your divergent way of thinking will rise, and there will be a reduction in your convergent way of thinking. You will experience a new change in the life that you are living and the one you will live after that. It is an incredible combination, but you will need expertise guide when you are preparing. Not prepare on your own since it can be dangerous.

CHAPTER 10
Controversies Around Ayahuasca

The drug ayahuasca has seen a rise in its popularity across the globe. It is because it has attracted several people interest. This has created seen several controversies over the years because of its popularity among people. The major attraction for people to ayahuasca is because they want to experience a certain form of awakening. Several questions have been raised about the practice of the drug. The major interest in this matter has taken a massive shift to the city of Iquitos. This a city found in the Peruvian rainforest which is a tourist attraction center. Several tourists are reported to be purchasing several cups of ayahuasca and taking them without any form of supervision.

Several deaths have been reported because of the unsupervised use of this drug. It is astonishing because the numbers of deaths associated with ayahuasca tends to rise nearly every year. This is despite the stimulant having several advantages poised on it. The deaths caused by ayahuasca have been reported several times and documented by the media. This is not supposed to be a discouraging factor for an individual interested in the brew. It is because it has been scientifically proven to have myriad advantages on an individual's mental health. There are several people who still visit the centers from the years of the 1920s. Most of the people who have had these visits and experience tend to have positive affirmations despite the presence of controversies around the plant. The highlighted controversies will be able to give an individual with in-depth insight into what really transpired and the relation to ayahuasca.

Reported Cases That Were Controversial
Case1: Motorcycle Accident

A British backpacker known as Mr. Henry Miller passed in the year 2014. This death incidence occurred in South America in a country known as Columbia. An amount of fifty dollars was paid by Mr Henry to give him a chance to participate in a ceremony entailing ayahuasca. The ceremony he aimed to partake in was advertised by his hostel and to be held in a certain lodge. There were several reports that were made by people who had witnessed him at the organized event. The reports from the witness stated that he was seen struggling and he later fell to a semi-unconscious state while in the ceremony. It was reported that the people who were in charge of the ceremony were not able to revive him.

However, it was later found out that Mr. Henry had died because of a different cause. It was established that he had died from an injury sustained on the head. The injury was because of a motorcycle accident he had encountered in the ceremony. The accident happened because of the incompetence by people who were running the ceremony. They were attempting to rush him to the hospital when he fell into the unconscious state. During his transportation, he fell off resulting him hitting his head really bad. This was the major cause of Mr Henry Miller's demise.

There are various things that go on in the tourism hub of ayahuasca which is Iquitos. The increasing impact of ayahuasca has had across the globe has seen the development of ayahuasca trade in a town known for heavy rubber trade. Ayahuasca vine jewelry, diets, and the arts are being sold. However, most tourists prefer to participate in ayahuasca ceremonies. Several centers have been set aside to make this process a success. This is because the product has been able to report success in helping people deal with several mental states. The therapeutic qualities it posses are healing of depression, anxiety, and several mental problems.

Case 2: Tobacco Poisoning

There was a reported death of a New Zealander in the year 2015. He was known as Mathew Dawson who as twenty-four years of age. His demise also occurred in a certain ayahuasca center in the region of Iquitos. The larger group of media reported globally with their headlines stating of his death being caused by ayahuasca. However, there was a small print of media that reported his death having a different cause. It was printed of his death to be caused by a tobacco purge. Tobacco is widely termed as a banned substance in several European countries because of its adverse effects on an individual's health. However, this is not the same case in Peru. It is because it is described as the master teacher plant in the traditions of the shaman in Peru.

Tobacco is widely smoked in the Peruvian regions. It is famously smoked as mapacho while in cigarette form in ayahuasca ceremonies. The practice is done because of a widely known reason of protecting the space. There is another form which ayahuasca is used in this region of the world. The second form is known as purgante in the local language or as purgative form in English. This form entails the tobacco is soaked in water for a couple of hours. It is then followed by individual drinking the substance which is supposed to trigger an individual to vomit. The process is always known as a cleansing ritual.

There was an intriguing even that was going on during the time Mr. Mathew died. Tobacco purges were being given to people during this time. The levels of these purges being safe are always high. However, there are certain cases these substances can result in an individual experiencing nicotine poisoning. Nicotine poisoning has adverse effects because it makes a person's organs to shut which can result in a person dying. This was a similar case to Mathew who was seen to be in great discomfort after he took the substance. He was in a great amount of physical discomfort because of the ingestion. He was witnessed screaming of being in so much pain and he later died because of a heart attack.

The proper usage of tobacco requires an individual working with a person with expertise on the substance. This is a skill that very few of the shamans who do their job with people interested in ayahuasca do not possess. There have been rising completion of the drug because of the increase in people who consume it. The competition is so stiff that it has seen several participants of ayahuasca product interested in outdoing each other. Some centers have gone to a different length of offering drugs that shamans do not have experience on how to handle the substance.

There are two plants that are on the rise of their usage. The plants are psychotropic cactus San Pedro and Oje. There are used for cleansing when ingested in their purgative form which is similar to the process used in the tobacco plant. They are very dangerous plants if an individual does not handle them with great caution. It is because Mr. Mathew was attended to by facilitators who not experienced as the shaman was watching a television set. The situation that befell Mathew is very sad because tobacco has the potential of affecting up to thirty percent of the world population. This is a controversy that has greatly surrounded the plant of ayahuasca.

Case 3: Murder

The death incidence in Iquitos that received massive media concentration was that of a Briton. The international media was quick to highlight the death of the twenty-four-year-old known as Unais Gomez. He was murdered by Joshua Stevens who was a Canadian. Both of these men were participants of an ayahuasca ceremony that was organized. These happening occurred in the year 2015. There were massive forms of propaganda that were spread over the incidence. The most fallacious information spread to people was that Mr. Stevens killed Mr. Gomez because of what was determined as a bad trip. The bad trip was characterized by Mr. Stevens experiencing visions that depicted Mr. Gomez having intercourse with his wife. The propaganda spread had infidelity visions as the cause of Mr. Gomez's death.

It was believed that Mr. Stevens had taken some ayahuasca substance that made him experience such hallucinations. There were toxicology tests that were conducted on Mr. Stevens after being apprehended. These tests were able to discover that the blood of Stevens did not have any form of ayahuasca content in him during the moments he stabbed Gomez. He pleaded his case to committing the act out of self-defense. These claims by Mr. Stevens were backed by a witness who confirmed Steven's story. The events were that Stevens had been allowed to conduct the ayahuasca ceremony that night in his room which was a private ceremony. Gomez later left the ceremony organized by a small group and headed to Stevens' room where he did attack him. Gomez was termed to seem possessed and it was very difficult for anyone to control him. The confrontation between the two men went to the kitchen. This was where Mr. Stevens picked up the knife and stabbed Mr. Gomez because he feared for his life.

Something that could be noted with an inner eye was that the group was not taken great care of. This is because it is very strange that the tourists were allowed to carry out such a ceremony without any help or supervision. It goes to be a very endangering situation when a participant in the ceremony is left to leave the group without the scrutiny of a shaman. The villagers who witnessed the occurrence termed the situation as Gomez to have been possessed by a demonic spirit. It is understood that the great power possessed by a shaman who was not present has the potential of combating and keeping out evil forces.

There are people who understand the situation that befell Gomez to be a psychotic state. This has the possibility of twisting the story to Gomez to be the one at fault because of his state. However, there were several findings of the information were done which revealed an interesting fact. It exposed that Gomez was not in a good mental state during the time of the unfolding. The situation did not make it safe for Gomez to drink ayahuasca. It is even discouraged for any individual to drink any medicinal plant that is described as psychoactive. There is one reason that also contributed to the death of Mr. Gomez. The center that allowed the group to organize the event did not receive past medical information about Mr. Gomez which could be used to stop the demise.

Case 4: Post-Ceremony Fatality

A Californian traveler was found dead in the year 2016 in the month of December. The thirty-eight-year-old found dead in the morning was known as Alfonso Geovanni D'Rose. His body was discovered in ayahuasca town in his room after attending an ayahuasca ceremony. The information given out by the shaman was that Mr Alfonso did not feel the impacts of the ayahuasca plant. He was then allowed to go back to his room with the permission of the shamans. This would culminate the end of his participation in the ceremony. The information about this occurrence could be described as little.

The little information pertaining to Mr. Alfonso's death was that he was found curled in his bathroom at a section opposite the toilet. There are several possibilities that were explored by people who were interested in the case. Some had the angle of reasoning that the effects of ayahuasca had made him pass on. It was because of the evident puke beside him. Other people went a notch hire to saying that maybe he ingested another substance such as sleeping pills. Mixing of the traditional and manufactured drug is an act that is greatly discouraged because of the impacts the two substances can make an individual go through.

The possibility of there being a medical event that was unforeseen was one thing that made sense to several people. This does not have to mean it's the icing of the true reason for the occurrence. However, it is a depiction of what can go wrong when an individual does not have the guide of the shaman in the process of ayahuasca intake.

SUMMARY OF THE BOOK

It has become a common phenomenon for people to travel to foreign destinations. One of the reasons is for them to have a taste of experience ayahuasca brings to an individual. It is a brew that is responsible for several psychotic functions. Several people have been keen on focusing on the immediate effects it brings. Several types of research have been conducted by scientists on the brew and its advantages have been proved to be legitimate.

Ayahuasca is described as the vine brewed from leaves of a plant known as Psychotria virus and then combined with stalks of Banisteriopsis caapi. These are two major ingredients which can be added to increase its effectiveness. The drink was majorly used in the past years for religious functions by the Arizonian tribes. This brew is also used by communities based in North America and Brazil. The person who leads and guides the process of preparation and intake of ayahuasca is known as a shaman.

The major components of this brew are hallucinogens. The components that are high in hallucinogens are broken down in an individual's liver. The components have the potential of affecting an individual's nervous system because of the psychedelic strength in the brew. This makes an individual be in a mental state where he or she experiences hallucinations, euphoria and out of body situations.

There are several activities that an individual is warned from before engaging in the ayahuasca ceremony. Some of the activities an individual is supposed to abstain from include smoking, sexual intercourse and taking of alcohol or caffeine. A person is supposed to take a vegetarian diet for an estimated period of two to three weeks. The process of taking a vegetative diet helps to clear an individual's body from toxins.

The ceremonies conducted by ayahuasca organizers tend to be conducted at night. They are ended when the effects of ayahuasca have worn out on people. The ceremony tends to commence after blessings by the shaman. The effects of ayahuasca are seen after an estimated time of twenty to sixty minutes. The effects can last from a varied period of two to six hours which is dependant on the dosage an individual has had. There are several effects that the substance has which include diarrhea and vomiting. These are considered as normal side effects of the substance. There are people who experience anxiety, panic or enlightened.

There are several people who have taken the brew and given out positive feedback. Some of these impacts have been long term and life-changing. It is because of the impact the brew has on an individual's neurological system. Scientific studies show that the brew contains neurorestorative and neuroprotective qualities in it which are key in the brain functioning. The stimulant is also very important to an individual who is seeking to improve his or her psychological well being. It is because ayahuasca improves an individual's mental awareness and general mental well being of a person. It has also helped in treating post-traumatic disorders, anxiety, and depression. There are controversies over this stimulant but the success outweighs them.

THANK YOU

Thank you for taking the time to read this book.
By now, you are supposed to have a good understanding of what ayahuasca is. The world has become a small global village where several things are unearthed every day in any location. Mental health is very important to an individual's life. The combination of the two factors of the world being a small village and the importance of mental health are what you have found to be the reason for the rapid increase in ayahuasca usage across the globe.
At this point, your mind has been educated on how the substance works. One is able to know of the two main components of the brew and the reason that the ancient drug was used. It is important for you to remember the process being very risky. There are adverse occurrences that can happen if an individual does not have guidance and help from a shaman. The education about diarrhea and voting being common side effects are pieces of information that can help you not to fall into a panic mode when you encounter them when taking ayahuasca.
Remember that it is important to always have both advantages and disadvantages of ayahuasca at your fingertips. You are able to recall that the disadvantages of this substance fall under the side effects they possess. However, the advantages outweigh the disadvantages. They have been proven to be legitimate and have the potential to have long term effects. You are educated about the controversies involving the substance the factual truth in them.

DESCRIPTION

What is Ayahuasca? What could be the origin? How does one prepare? What is it used for? How does one administer Ayahuasca traditionally? Does it have any effects on our body? What is the science behind ayahuasca? Does it have any controversy?

Ayahuasca can be described as a brew that is made from mixing some ingredients with banisteriopsis. The main reason this brew is prepared is that it will be used for cleansing in the traditional ceremonies. It is even used as a sacrament because they felt that there was a spiritual connection and they treasured it so much. While in the modern days it used to heal those with mental illness and those who are sick physically. For those who have tried using it some have registered positive results yet for others, they were affected negatively by the brew. For those who are using it, they should do that with a lot of caution because ayahuasca has the side effects on the body. The side effects are diarrhea, vomiting and it also causes an increase in the heartbeat rate in other people.

It can be prepared by boiling the banisteriopsis with leaves of Psychotria Viridis and diplopterys cabrerana and many other leaves. The taste will vary because of the different leaves used. The quality of the brew will depend on the kind of ingredients used plus if the right procedure was followed. The process will take seven hours or even more than that. The reason why the brewing process will take longer is that the mixture of the vine and the leaves are left to boil till half the pot. From there the brew will be ready for consumption.

That is the reason most tourists will travel to the west part of African countries to try to look for ayahuasca so that they can be used as a medicine. This tourist needs to find out the legit healers for them to get the correct information before they proceed to take the medication. It is good to obtain the correct information from the correct source. It will help you know the positive effects of the product plus the negative effects. From there you will way and see what to go for.

The main goal of this book is to understand what Ayahuasca is, the history behind the existence of this brew, and the reason why we have it...

In this book you'll learn:
- What is Ayahuasca?
- The Origin of Ayahuasca
- History of Ayahuasca and how it became known in the West.
- How to Make and Prepare Ayahuasca
- What Ayahuasca is Used For
- How Ayahuasca is Traditionally Administered
- Different Uses of Ayahuasca and Why One Would Choose a Certain Use
- The science Behind Ayahuasca

- Effects of Ayahuasca in the Body
- Controversy Around Ayahuasca

Would you like to learn more about Ayahuasca?

Purchase this book today and equip yourself with the right knowledge about ayahuasca and the history behind it!

www.ingramcontent.com/pod-product-compliance
Lightning Source LLC
Chambersburg PA
CBHW071510070526
44578CB00001B/498